GET HEALTHY, ST

GET HEALTHY, STAY HEALTHY

The Essential Guide to Food, Life and Love

Laura Ackerman
with Barbara Davidson

Foreword by Jan de Vries

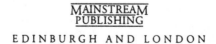

MAINSTREAM
PUBLISHING

EDINBURGH AND LONDON

First published in Great Britain in 1999 by
MAINSTREAM PUBLISHING COMPANY (EDINBURGH) LTD
7 Albany Street
Edinburgh EH1 3UG

ISBN 1 84018 203 2

A CIP catalogue record for this book is available from the
British Library

Typeset in Sabon
Printed and bound in Finland by WSOY

Contents

Foreword

It is with the greatest interest that I have read Laura Ackerman's book on how to get healthy and stay healthy.

Having known Laura both as a patient and as a friend for a very long time, I have always admired her great zeal and desire to help others. It was due to this desire that she branched out into the area of nutritional health, where she has since helped many people through her work. She writes with great conviction on how we can improve our health, covering subjects such as diet and remedies, including the role of vitamins, minerals and trace elements. She wrote this book so that she could share her wealth of experience and knowledge in order to help others, and I am sure that her readers will find the advice contained in these pages invaluable.

Laura has often discussed with me the philosophies which the late Dr Alfred Vogel and I developed while working together for over forty years. Laura's enthusiasm and passion for learning more about the role played by nature in maintaining our health is always delightful to behold. In this book she explains that by providing the correct conditions for the body and by supplying it with the necessary nutrition, it is possible to reactivate the body's own regeneration system. In this way, it is possible to treat and overcome many different ailments.

During the many years that I have spent working within the field of complementary medicine, I have endorsed the message that prevention is better than cure. In the same way, Laura has emphasised in her book that it is important not only to treat the obvious symptoms of illness, as conventional medicine would do, but that we also have to learn to look for the causes of these symptoms and therefore find a cure for the source of the illness. There is no point in getting rid of an ache or a particular sensitivity in the body if we are unable to eliminate the cause. In order to do this, it is necessary to recognise which factors have contributed to the illness.

I am convinced that this book will play a very important role in guiding and educating people not only in recovering fully from ill health, but also in maintaining their health at its maximum potential.

Jan de Vries, DHo.med, Do,
MRO, NDMRN, DAcMBAcA

About the author

I was born an optimist, a Leo and redheaded, and nothing much has changed except for the appearance of a few grey hairs. Although there was only my brother Jim and me in our family, my mother was the youngest of ten children and we were always surrounded by our cousins, aunts and uncles. Every Saturday and Sunday evening the family would gather at my grandmother's house and usually someone would offer to entertain us with a song or a story or a poem. Actually, poem isn't the right word – it was always more of a funny, rhyming story which could go on for 20 verses and always caused great hilarity. Everyone in the family had their favourite party piece and I was encouraged to have mine. I was always pleased when it was my turn to sing and dance because, yes, I did both. Looking back, this was such a good lesson. It encouraged me to be outgoing and sing for my supper. I still love to entertain, but nowadays I restrict myself to cooking and giving parties – although I must admit it's seventh heaven to be able to sing and dance with my two-year-old grandson.

I developed my passion for health and nutrition when I lived for four years in California, and when I returned to live in Scotland at the age of 22 I brought back with me all the health books I could carry. My passion and commitment has grown throughout the years; what might have seemed an optional extra interest at that time is now to me essential for health.

I have been married and divorced and have lived abroad and all these experiences and relationships have moulded me and had an effect on my health and strength. I would say I have lived a full and eventful life.

This past year has been the hardest of my life. My husband, Rob Logan, died in a climbing accident in May 1998 and the loss and shock of that is still with me.

Being a mother to Barbara has been the best part of my life. My brother Jim calls me a hands-on mother and now it's wonderful to be a hands-on grandmother, too, because I also get time off for good behaviour – or, as I call it, rest and relaxation.

I have lived with mental illness in my close family and have witnessed what unhappiness and emptiness can do to a person and to everyone around them. I know that physical and mental health do go together and that so often the life that we live and choose as adults has much to do with the way we were treated as children. I think it is healthy to apportion blame; it's important to understand that as adults we must accept responsibility and as parents we must be aware of the effects that our behaviour has on our children. To anyone who wants to take this further, may I suggest you read Alice Miller's *The Drama of the Gifted Child*.

I have learned that how we live, what we eat and how we feel when we eat is a serious business, but that few of us take it seriously enough. It seems that as a nation we are cooking less and enjoying our food less, but at the same time watching more and more cookery programmes on television. It's right that chefs should become stars because they are giving us what we need and recognise to be important to us. They are proud to admit they will slave over a hot stove to give us a few delicious mouthfuls.

We can't separate our hearts and our heads from our stomach and digestion because everything within us, I believe, is connected. There is little point giving advice on food and dietary supplements to someone whose life is in turmoil, and expect to see an improvement in their health. That simply won't happen.

In spite of everything I have experienced, I still expect good things to happen. I could have called this book *An Optimist's Guide to Health* because that's what it is. I want you to read this book and enjoy it and, whether you follow some of my recommendations, or just a few of the ideas I suggest, or even none at all, I want you to feel good about yourself and enjoy your life.

Best wishes for your good health.

Laura Ackerman
Glasgow
February 1999

Barbara Davidson BSc is Laura Ackerman's daughter and has benefited from having a healthy upbringing. Educated in Edinburgh and Dundee, she has a degree in psychology and is a trained teacher. Happily married, she is now the proud mother of a beautiful baby boy.

Preface

My aim in this book is to show how your choice of foods, how you eat them, where you eat them and how you feel when you eat them all have a huge effect on your weight.

If there wasn't enough consideration given to your needs and wants when you were young and you had to eat the food you were given and were not allowed to choose, it may be that as you grew older you lost touch with your own feelings as to what you wanted and what was good for your body.

It may have been that when you were young you felt there wasn't enough food for you. Maybe your family was large or couldn't afford to spend a lot of money on food, or perhaps you went to boarding school and there wasn't enough food to go round. Or it may have been the case that when food was available you simply ate whatever you could, quickly, to make sure you got your share. This way of eating may have continued long after your original circumstances had changed.

Perhaps when you were young you were forced to clear your plate and eat food you didn't want or like. It may have been your mother pleading with you to eat a little more because she had gone to a lot of trouble cooking for you, or your father insisting that wasting food was a disgrace and a sign you were ungrateful. Maybe your family gave you three large meals a day and you would have preferred six smaller meals or snacks a day, or perhaps your mother was a terrible cook and everything she made was heavy and tasteless but you had to eat it even though you didn't enjoy it. It may have been that you were living in a tense, unhappy family and every mealtime was just misery and all you wanted to do was eat as fast as you could and leave the table so you could disappear with your books, games or friends.

Maybe you didn't eat a balanced diet when you were growing up. Your meals may have lacked variety so you developed a lot of likes and dislikes and wouldn't even try many foods. It's hard to get enough nourishment and vitamins when you restrict yourself to just a few foods all the time.

If you were emotionally cajoled or threatened to clear your plate and punished if you didn't, or if your pleas for more food were ignored, you may have continued this way of eating into adulthood. You may be aware today sub-consciously that you eat too fast, that you must always clear your plate and that you often have a heavy stomach, indigestion or discomfort afterwards.

All these things, which many, many people experience, can have a tremendous effect on your eating habits today. The state of your health now is likely to have been greatly influenced by your upbringing.

This book looks at some of the most important aspects of a woman's life – menstrual problems, pregnancy, child-rearing and the menopause – as well as at a host of other areas, and offers nutritional advice and sensible suggestions to overcome the difficulties we all face in our daily lives. For example, I discuss how emotions and thoughts can affect weight. There are aspects of your personality which developed in your childhood and these traits can greatly influence your physical health as well as your mental health. Not enough consideration is given to how your own nature controls and affects your digestive system. Some people, regardless of how much they try to watch what they eat, are in the grip of an emotional need for food or are unable to eliminate what they eat.

I explain how much of the discomfort suffered during the menstrual cycle can be traced to poor elimination and a lack of essential minerals. I recommend the necessary supplements to relax the body and muscles, give a feeling of well-being and stop mood swings.

I advise on how to improve your health in the expectation of becoming pregnant, suggesting ways to get your body into the best possible condition by eating the best foods available, taking all the appropriate supplements and organising your life so you can reduce any stresses, mental or physical, as much as possible.

I make suggestions to eliminate some of the unpleasant side-effects of pregnancy, such as morning sickness, bloating and tiredness. Many women worry about gaining excess weight during pregnancy and being unable to lose it after the birth, so I give advice for before and during pregnancy to produce not only a healthier baby but also a healthier and fitter mother, too.

I offer suggestions on how to feed and care for your baby so that he or she can get the best possible start in life. By looking at different ways of feeding your baby, I show how to prevent your child experiencing many of the so-called everyday problems of colic, wind, constipation and dry skin, making sure yours is not a crying, unsettled baby.

I discuss the symptoms and discomfort associated with the menopause – weight gain, hot flushes, tender breasts, sore joints and dry skin and many more – and suggest natural alternatives to hormone replacement therapy.

There comes a point in most people's lives when they look in the mirror and realise they are not as young as they once were. They might look tired and worn out and not even recognise their own reflection. I advise on rejuvenation and how to make the best of what you have in terms of the state of your physical and emotional health.

In addition to the above, the book also gives more general advice relating to food and nutrition. For example, I explain why your appetite and sugar craving and storing of excess weight are all controlled by your blood-sugar level. A fluctuating BSL can result in erratic eating habits and patterns which make it very hard to lose weight. I explain how we can balance this and keep the BSL steady so that weight will be lost, cravings will disappear, and you will never yo-yo diet again.

Any discomfort such as bloating, burping, heartburn, wind, indigestion or pain can be caused by eating hard-to-digest foods and eating them too quickly. The best way to be slender and healthy is to eat health-giving foods and it's worth making the effort to vary your diet. Eating is not simply a way to get rid of your hunger; it should be a relaxing and enjoyable experience that will also satisfy your body's need for nutrition. Eating a better, more varied diet should become part of your life. Vitamins and minerals are an extra form of food, and a lack of vitamins can keep you overweight.

I have provided 14 days' worth of menus to give you a balanced diet with enough protein, carbohydrate, fruit and vegetables to improve your health, increase your energy and help you stay slender.

Introduction

This book represents my own personal feelings and experiences on health. I hope you will find it a friendly, practical, easy-to-read guide to help you deal with a selection of problems that we all come across in our lives. I have learnt so much from my clients and I have watched them change into healthier, more vital people with fewer problems. Good health is such a precious thing. Often we only appreciate how fragile it is when we come close to losing it – or when we lose sight of what good health should be.

I do believe it is easy for you to lose weight and improve your health at the same time. If you have struggled with your weight so far, you will find it hard to believe me. So far everything in your experience has told you that it's difficult to lose weight. That's just not true. I'll explain the causes of weight gain, how your body is affected and what steps you have to take to lose the weight. I'm going to keep it as simple as possible and hopefully answer your questions as I go along. I'll explain how to improve your health so you can live the life you want to live and be the person you want to be. This is quite a task but I believe I have the knowledge and the experience to help you change your life if you really want to. It's up to you. You can read the book and then decide if you want to take the easy and simple-to-follow steps to make the difference. This book is not simply about losing weight: a healthy body will not store excess weight but will be vibrant, vital and looking for life.

Many of us at some time in our lives want to lose weight. Through my work as a health and diet consultant within my health food business I have helped many people successfully lose weight and improve their health at the same time. This is, I hope, a simple guide to help *you* lose weight easily. It may be that you want to lose a few pounds or a couple of stone. Either way, by following these simple steps it should be easy for you to achieve your optimum weight and get the best you can out of life.

Frequently whilst advising people on weight loss I have found that my clients feel they have to apologise for being overweight. Often they don't expect me to believe them when they tell me that they feel they don't overeat. They believe they eat an average amount – perhaps even less than their family or friends – and yet their weight steadily increases. I begin by reassuring them that for the majority of people overeating is not the problem – it's faulty digestion that is to blame. Once we discover what is hindering healthy digestion we can start to make improvements to boost health and lose weight at the same time.

Here are five of the main reasons why people find it hard to lose weight:

+ the body not cleansing
+ poor digestion
+ a lack of vitamins or minerals
+ eating hard-to-digest food
+ lack of simple exercise

Let me show you the easy way to weight loss and good health. I will lead you step by step through the whole process, beginning by showing you how to cleanse and detoxify your body. Next, I will discuss the best foods to eat and those to avoid, providing sample menus and simple recipes for easy-to-cook dishes. I will show you how to stop sugar cravings and forget yo-yo dieting forever. I will give you my advice on what we call 'women's health' which includes conceiving, pregnancy care and the first few months of motherhood. As my daughter is a new mother, I am acutely aware of what a happy and also traumatic time this can be and how important it is for her to keep up her strength and energy. The secret, of course, is to be prepared and save your energy because once it's gone, it's ten times harder for you to get it back.

This book also contains a chapter on vitality for men to encourage your husband or partner to take better care of himself and join you in good health – it's no good if you are filled with energy and health and wanting to dance until dawn if your beloved is asleep in his chair before the *Nine O'Clock News*.

I'll explain how your own nature, and your past and present relationships influence your appetite and your weight.

I want to make it clear that this book can change your life!

Throughout the book the nutritional advice is combined with practical tips for health, and I'll always add a boost of confidence at the same time. I will explain my recommendations step by step, so this book will show you how to improve your health and lose weight, and allow you to work at your own pace.

If you are only a few pounds overweight it's simple to get back on an even keel using the advice in this book. If your health is poor and you are also overweight you may think that by losing weight you will get your health back. It is like that for some people but not for all. Your body may be overweight *because* your health is poor. You may have to improve your health before you are able to lose weight. In either case vitamins will help.

Taking the right vitamins can help all your problems and give you vitality. But how do you find out which ones you need? Begin with my suggested supplements and then listen to your body. If you are less tired or your joints feel easier or if the symptoms you have been suffering begin to ease off or disappear then you know you are on the right track. Keep going – increase the amount of pills you are taking or find the equivalent food that's loaded with the vitamin you need. Drink organic carrot juice instead of taking betacarotene, for example. Eat more fruit instead of taking vitamin C, and replace calcium and magnesium with more organic root vegetables.

Your own personal outlook on life

Is your cup half empty or half full? Your answer to this question reveals a lot about you and the life you have. Optimists will always say 'half full'. Just as many things go wrong for them and they have just as many problems and challenges to face as pessimists, but it's their attitude that makes the difference. Whenever Scarlett O'Hara in *Gone with the Wind* was faced with a problem she always said, 'I'll think about that tomorrow,' which could be another way of saying, 'I'll concentrate on everything good now and worry about my problems later.'

Optimists can also seem to have bad memories! No matter what has gone wrong for them in the past and how much trouble, hassle or money it has cost them, if you give them a new idea or direction, off they'll go like a playful puppy. If someone tries to remind them what happened before, they won't listen. It will be different this time, they say, this will be great, super, easy, happy ending. I have to declare that I am an optimist. I couldn't advise on health if I wasn't. No matter what problems my clients have, I always feel something can be done to help them. There has been a lot of research carried out which proves your attitude to life can affect your health, for good or bad. By checking your psychological profile it's even possible to work out in advance which illnesses you may be pre-disposed to.

When my clients consult me about their health, I attempt to make things as clear and as simple as possible for them. I take time to explain what I think their body is lacking in terms of nutrients; I suggest certain changes to their diet and try to predict the positive effects they will feel. In this way I share knowledge with them and provide pointers so they can see their health improving and be aware of the reasons behind the improvement. I always check that they have understood my explanation and I ask if they will follow my recommendations. They must promise me and themselves they will do it.

Is it harder on your health if you are a pessimist? I would say so. If you are tense, anxious and always expecting something to go wrong then naturally your brain will be sending the signal 'trouble ahead, get ready for action'. It is flight or fight. Your body is on constant alert and this is enough to wear anyone down quickly. Think how exhausted you feel after 20 minutes under obvious stress like sitting a driving test, making a court appearance or asking for a pay-rise. We are all aware of these high levels of tension at times, but many people unconsciously or subconsciously cause themselves unnecessary stress by looking for problems where there are none.

Your mental attitude to life does affect your physical state. It is clear that an optimistic person with a positive outlook will be expecting good things to happen and will be less tense as a result. Someone with a fearful or negative attitude will be holding their body more tensely and this tension can act as a barrier to an improvement in health. It is perhaps also true to say that a pessimist will be more concerned about the state of their health than an optimistic person. A large proportion of my clients are pessimists – perhaps as many as 90 per cent of them. It may be that pessimists heavily outnumber optimists in life generally. I give a huge amount of positive encouragement to all my pessimistic clients, of course. It is in my nature to be this way. It can be hard and a drain on my energy but I notice that most people require coaxing and support to persevere with improving their health. This is why I give individual, one-to-one consultations at my practice.

I have learned – and continue to learn – so much from my clients. I am very grateful to every one of them for opening up to me. During a consultation, we look for the root of the problem and this can often require quite a lot of discussion about the past. Not all health difficulties have hidden causes, however. It seems to me there are only two types of people – givers and takers.

It's surprising how many people think they are takers when they are in fact givers. Make allowances for yourself. Don't compare yourself to anyone. We are all different and have abilities to cope with different things in our lives.

Is your past making you sick?

One woman came to me suffering from great anxiety and couldn't find any reason for it – she had good health, a good husband, happy children and no obvious reason for her misery. She felt she was an ungrateful person as she couldn't enjoy her life. We discovered that, as the youngest of a large family, she was the one who stopped family arguments and spent as much time as possible at home keeping the peace. Twenty years later, the anxiety was still there although the circumstances were totally different.

Some of our clients won't take responsibility for their own health. When they hand over money for a consultation or pills it is as if they are handing over the responsibility for their health. One man very much wanted to lose weight and when we discussed his diet it became clear that he was living on microwaved convenience food and didn't like fruit and vegetables. I advised a cleansing programme and a course of nutrients to rebuild his health. Within a month he looked like a different person – clear skin, thicker hair, brighter eyes and less jumpy. He hadn't lost any weight during this time, however, and although he admitted there may have been some slight improvement in his health he wouldn't really believe anything was working until he saw it on the scales. Most people will improve their diet when they start to see a change in their health. When they realise that it is possible to improve their health they open up to new ideas.

As I mentioned, a great number of my clients have required a huge amount of support and encouragement as they attempt the task of improving their health. I know that those who believe they are going to recover or regain good health soon do actually achieve that state much more quickly than someone who is reluctant to believe the good news. This is a big part of the reason I decided to write this book – I want more people to believe that it is possible to feel physically and mentally well. It is such a source of satisfaction for me to see clients looking and feeling healthier. It is why I enjoy what I do. I know I am helping people to improve their lives.

How we perceive ourselves to be has a huge effect on how we actually are. Our idea of self and what we are affects so many areas of our lives. I remember a school-friend of mine who, when I would say, 'Your hair looks lovely today,' would reply, 'What was wrong with it yesterday?' My compliments and admiration fell on deaf ears. She didn't see what I saw. She so needed to be admired and yet she rebuffed all praise. She married a man who loved her and thought her beautiful in every way, and she was. After a short honeymoon period, she refused to accept his compliments and at the same time allowed herself to become plain and dowdy. She grew into what she saw in the mirror of her head.

It is important to be aware of how your mental attitude can affect your physical health. I believe that in time your thoughts will show on your body.

Why do I suffer after eating?

1

Let us begin by discussing internal cleansing. What may appear to you to be a problem of weight retention could simply be a problem with elimination. When I speak about healthy cleansing and elimination, it simply means you are eating foods you can digest; these are then being processed easily through your stomach and the waste products from these foods will then be eliminated from your bowels regularly every day. If you are not cleansing and eliminating every day you could suffer from a host of symptoms such as a general feeling of tiredness, cold hands and feet, varicose veins, thyroid problems, lacklustre skin, dandruff or athlete's foot – and, of course, weight gain. One peculiar symptom of indigestion may be a lack of appetite or even the opposite – finding you constantly want to eat because you never feel full or satisfied.

What is a cleansing diet?

A cleansing diet would be a 48-hour period where you would avoid alcohol, tea and coffee and convenience or fast foods. It is simple and easy for your body to cope with. You would have light home-made soups without cream, as well as simple foods and as much fresh fruit, salads and vegetables as you would enjoy. You still need protein for a balanced diet so I would recommend dishes such as poached eggs, grilled fish and roast chicken.

It would also help you to have as much rest and relaxation as possible (unplug the phone!). Some people have told me they don't feel they have time to detox. It may seem like something that requires effort when in fact detoxing at a particularly busy or stressful time can really help. Don't tell yourself you'll wait till you're relaxed before you attempt a period of cleansing – that may never happen – and when you're feeling tense your digestive system is under pressure anyway so simple foods would help.

For most of us, changes to our health take place over a period of months or even years and because of that we accept how we are today as normal. When I ask a client, 'When did you last feel great?', they usually have to think hard before they can answer. It's not normal or a sign of good health to have bad circulation where your hands and feet are always cold. Cellulite, usually on your thighs, and sometimes showing up as white fatty tissue in the skin beneath your eyes, is a sign your body is not eliminating well. Tender breasts and excessive swelling in your stomach before your period is another sign of slow elimination. Varicose veins anywhere in your body again means your system is not emptying properly. Likewise, liver spots on your hands, arms or face are a good indicator. Your liver cannot cope with the constant reprocessing of the same old waste that keeps going round and round and doesn't leave! Thankfully your liver can repair and renew itself if we start cleansing your body and then take a course of herbs until the liver spots start to fade. (The two herbs I recommend the most for liver repair are St John's Wort or Milk Thistle.)

Skin-brushing can also be an extra help when you are cleansing, and I would recommend that you try it once a week. Buy a soft-bristle brush and begin by lightly brushing your skin. Work in circles in a clockwise direction and always towards your heart. Skin-brushing stimulates circulation so we should encourage the flow of blood *towards*

25

the heart. You could also exfoliate your skin by using a face-cloth which has been rinsed in warm water with a handful of sea salt added. Dead Sea mineral salts are worth finding. Massaging your body this way will remove dead skin cells and allow your body to breathe, at the same time stimulating your system to eliminate waste. Rinse your skin, towel it dry and then massage in either almond, avocado, grape-seed or jojoba oil. Remember your skin is a major organ in your body and it plays an important role in elimination.

Identifying poor digestion

I begin by advising my clients to follow my advice on cleansing and then ask them questions to assess the state of their digestion. When I ask if they suffer from indigestion, they usually answer no – probably because most people relate indigestion to the burning sensation of heartburn, and that is one symptom they may not be experiencing. When I ask the following questions, however, the answers usually reveal that digestion is the problem:

+ Do you wake up tired in the morning?
+ Do you suffer from bloating after meals?
+ Do your clothes get tighter round the waist as the day goes on?

Very frequently the answer is yes to all three. These are all signs of indigestion and the next step is to find the cause.

Indigestion

Let us consider the following questions to reveal more about your digestion:

- Do you feel hungover after only a few drinks?
- Could you happily skip breakfast in the morning?
- Do you tend to put on weight more round the middle than anywhere else, making your body shape more apple than pear?
- Do you have prematurely grey hair for your age?

Answering yes to any of these questions can be a sign of poor or slow digestion.

There are many different ways of improving your digestion and losing excess weight. Many of my clients feel their digestion clears up after a few days on a cleansing diet. I would suggest trying this diet and finding out more about your digestive system for a few days.

For some people it is simply the case that their indigestion is caused by eating their food too quickly. Chewing produces saliva which then releases digestive juices in your stomach, so that spending more time on each mouthful can help greatly.

For others, a lack of B vitamins can result in indigestion and taking a course of these vitamins can help relax you and thus aid digestion. I would also recommend a course of digestive enzymes which not only help you digest your food but also extract the nutrients so you can really get the best out of the food you eat. Many of my clients have been helped by these two simple steps of cleansing and taking digestive aids.

Mind and body combined

The ideal eating pattern for a healthy digestive system is to have a leisurely breakfast, a light nutritious lunch and a relaxed evening meal in the company of family and friends. Not many of us live that way. For most people it's a rush with a cup of coffee or cereal in the morning, a dash out for a sandwich at lunchtime or a business lunch where you are talking and eating at the same time with one eye on the clock. By the time you get home at night you are too tired to buy or cook wholesome food, so it's either a takeaway or a microwaved convenience meal. If you are so tired that you eat your meal either quickly or in front of the television, the food simply won't be digested. To make matters worse, going to bed quite soon after you've eaten means the food will lie in your stomach overnight, and when you wake in the morning you'll feel tired, sluggish and in no mood for breakfast.

The biggest task your body has all day is to digest your food. It can actually take up to 80 per cent of your daily energy simply to break down the food and extract the nutrients you require from it.

If we can't change your daily life and the pressure you are living under, what can we do to make it easier for your digestive system to cope? Well, first of all try to avoid eating a full meal when you're tired or in a rush or just going to bed. Eat the minimum amount possible. I would suggest you chew each mouthful twenty times, putting your cutlery down between mouthfuls.

Another thing which may help to make life easier for your digestion is to try food combining. The main thought behind food combining is to avoid eating protein and carbohydrates during the same meal. This means you would eat fish, chicken, meat, eggs or cheese (protein) alone, or you would eat starchy foods such as potatoes, rice, pasta and bread (carbohydrates) alone. This way of eating can make a major difference to your digestive system, one of the reasons being that food combining doesn't allow you to eat convenience foods and you have to stick to simple foods.

It's essential for good digestion to get enough oils every day and I usually recommend two tablespoons of virgin olive oil used either in cooking or on salads as a dressing with fresh lemon.

Dairy products

Food that is hard to digest makes the body's task even more difficult. Dairy products are often the main culprit. It takes a lot of enzymes and stomach acid to break down milk, cream, cheese and yoghurt. You need these enzymes in order for your body to extract the goodness from the food and to eliminate the waste. We are all encouraged to buy semi-skimmed and skimmed milk, but I believe we are better off with full-fat milk because all the enzymes necessary for digestion are already there in the milk fat. Many of us, especially people with fair hair, pale skin and blue eyes, lack these milk-digesting enzymes. This simply means we can't break down the milk protein and therefore we don't gain nutritionally from these foods. Because they are mostly undigested, the resulting waste can't be eliminated efficiently, and will stay too long inside us, adding to our weight gain.

So what happens to this waste? Our bodies try to help us by storing the extra waste where we may be able to expel it ourselves. This can show up as catarrh, resulting in bronchitis or sinusitis, and in this way we can blow our noses or cough the waste up. I never tire of saying: the body is so perfect it never makes a mistake. There is a good reason for all your symptoms and they are your body's way of trying to keep you as healthy as possible until it can find another method of solving the problem.

How is it possible that eating a little cheese or cream, perhaps just a few times a week, could keep you overweight? Well, let's say you sit down to a meal of fruit, and perhaps a piece of fish or chicken and vegetables. You enjoy it and your system feels good. The next day you have the same meal except this time you also have a creamy dessert or cheese to follow. Having the cream or cheese can be the equivalent of someone without enough milk-digesting enzymes eating a lump of candle wax. Hard to break down, it prevents all the food in the stomach being digested. This means that everything that's been eaten will lie there inside and nothing will be digested. The candle comparison may be a little extreme but what I'm trying to say is that if it's not digestible, it's not digestible, whatever it's called.

So all the food and the dairy products are lying in your stomach – what happens now? Your stomach extends and bloats and feels heavy and uncomfortable. You get heartburn or you want to burp all night long. You feel so tired you want to lie down but you can't, because you have lots more to do, so you go and have something to eat for energy and a pick-me-up and the weight gain and discomfort continue.

So some of us can't digest the milk protein in milk, cream, cheese and yoghurt and that's the problem. We can still eat butter as it contains fat only and has no protein and is therefore digestible.

Soya and tofu

For some people soya and tofu can be harder to digest than dairy products. Anyone who has ever tried to cook soya beans could vouch for this – they can take days to soften. It is common practice nowadays for many biscuits, cakes and breads to contain soya flour so it's worth checking labels or asking your local baker for a list of ingredients. These suggestions may sound overly cautious but I have

30

seen many people's health or weight problems diminish after a period of eating simpler, less-processed foods so I know it will help to avoid products containing soya if you can. This includes the soy sauce on your Chinese meal!

Chocolate

There is no reason to stop eating chocolate, as the best-tasting brands are naturally dairy-free. Most health-food stores, along with shops such as Oxfam, sell Green & Black's delicious dairy-free chocolate. Chocolate from other European countries tends to be higher in cocoa solids with less vegetable fat than your average British bar and lighter on your digestive system – so staying away from dairy products needn't be a punishment.

Easing digestion

Would you now consider reducing your intake of dairy products for a two-week period? This may lead to a feeling of lightness, ease in digestion and weight loss. If you notice any discomfort such as bloating or nasal congestion when you return to eating dairy products, you can always restrict or eliminate them if you want to. You may of course find that your health problems have been greatly helped by this change in diet. The next step for anyone still suffering from indigestion would be to eliminate or at least restrict starchy carbohydrates such as pasta, rice and potatoes. Try this for two weeks and see if it helps. You can still eat bread in the form of toast as this turns the starch into sugar and is easier to digest.

Over the past twenty years we have become conditioned into believing that a healthy diet is one that is low in fat and high in carbohydrates. I have found, however, that my clients are healthier and slimmer on a diet which is high in protein – in meat, fish, poultry, eggs and cheese – if they can digest it. I suggest this diet for a large number of my clients and it does seem to help. They tell me they feel more energetic and crave less sugar.

Recommended steps to weight loss

I am now going to lead you through a list of diet-supplement recommendations and advise you which products may be of help to you. Proceed as quickly or slowly as feels right to you.

Aloe Vera 25ml morning and night
Vitamin C 500mg morning and dinner
Vitamin B complex 50mg after each meal
Superdigestaway two before each meal
Spirulina one capsule after each meal
Vitamin E one 100iu capsule with best meal of the day
Betacarotene one 15mg capsule with best meal of the day

After five days I would expect you to feel lighter and aware of changes in your body for the better. It's hard to be more specific with reactions to Aloe Vera as it is such a wonderful product it seems to go directly to the part or organ of your body where it is most needed. Arthritis sufferers say Aloe Vera eases their joint pain. People with an itch or rash say it clears the problem in a few days. For slimmers it will cleanse and heal you internally.

We are going to add a good-quality naturally occurring multi-vitamin, Spirulina, which will encourage your body to work better. It will give you essential vitamins and minerals, including iron, in a form ready for assimilation.

This multi-vitamin will increase your energy and health.

Now add Vitamin E to your diet. In the past we were able to get enough Vitamin E naturally from our foods; nowadays, however, to give bread and cake a long shelf-life, it has been extracted from these foods. Add beta-carotene to your list, as you would have to eat an extremely large amount of carrots, yellow peppers, peaches, nectarines and apricots on a daily basis to get sufficient quantities. In my experience people who work at a computer screen have high demands for betacarotene in particular.

How long will you have to keep taking all these pills? The answer depends on how quickly your body responds, and how much weight you're trying to lose. I would suggest you follow my advice and take the supplements faithfully for one month, then stop taking them for a couple of days. This will let you know if there was any benefit while you were taking the pills. It may be that as you progress you would be more comfortable with this pattern. You yourself are the best judge of the best pace for you.

This is just some of the advice that I've been giving on weight loss and good health for the last twenty years. It's taken a lot of commitment on my part and much more from my clients for them to lose weight successfully. People who had heard of me by word of mouth would persevere with my diet suggestions, as they knew their friends had lost weight and become healthier by following my recommendations. They were hopeful they too would be successful – and they were! This is tried and tested advice.

How can I be slender as well as healthy?

2

There are many reasons why I consider it necessary to supplement our diet with vitamins to obtain enough nutrients. Thirty years ago the food that we ate would have been grown locally, picked and transported to our corner shops within a day. We would have chosen what we needed for the day, taken it home and cooked it. Many people now do their weekly shopping in a supermarket, buying foods that were picked perhaps six weeks earlier, that spent many days in transit and were kept in cold storage. We sometimes hear reports that apples we buy today may have been kept in cold storage for a whole year before being offered for sale and may lack the essential vitamins we need for health. Most of the fruit and vegetables that we eat were never allowed to sweeten on the vine and may never fully ripen. If we buy these fruits and vegetables from a display in a supermarket, they may have been sitting under bright light which in itself is enough to destroy many vitamins. During the course of a normal day they may also have been sprinkled several times with water by the supermarket staff to keep them looking shiny and attractive. The soil they come from can be over-farmed and many soil tests have shown a lack of the essential minerals that we need for health.

All this may sound as if I recommend avoiding fruit and vegetables. On the contrary, I advise eating a good amount of them – but be fussy and selective about what you buy. Be aware of what you are eating and of the benefits to your body. Look for the best quality fresh produce and, if you can, support any local greengrocer who is trying to supply good quality ingredients.

What to eat

Food should be packed with health and vitality. I've spent the last thirty years preparing, cooking and eating the best food I could find. I find cooking relaxing and it's my hobby, and I'm not suggesting that you do the same if you have different interests. But I have often been asked what I eat and if I have any advice on food – so here it is!

I buy locally whenever I can and I do not shop in super-markets unless I have no other alternative. I shop daily and buy organically grown produce wherever possible. It is more expensive but I would rather eat one organically grown apple than three commercially grown fruits. Organi-cally grown fruit and vegetables may not look as attractive and perfect as the commercially grown varieties. The dif-ference is in the taste and our bodies will thrive on the essential vitamins and minerals that they supply from their organic soil.

A comparison can be made with the roses we now buy from the florists. They are perfect in every way but they have no scent. We realise the flowers are lacking strength in some form and it must be the same with tasteless fruit and vegetables.

I buy from my local butcher and my local fishmonger and the same with the bread shop and cheese shop. I buy and eat a large variety of the freshest and best quality locally grown produce I can find. I go to a lot of trouble and effort but I think it is worth it – I have wonderful health and I also enjoy delicious meals. At the end of the book is a short list of all the people I buy from who have a mail-order service.

Everyone thrives better on fresh, wholesome foods and we do need a variety of them. After all, variety is the spice of life! There are at least 28 different fruits and more than 39 different vegetables and each one supplies a variety of different nutrients that are good for our health.

If you make the effort to cook good quality food you *will* feel the benefit. Your body needs enough nutrients or it simply cannot do all the work it has to do. If you don't give your body what it needs you should not be surprised if you feel run-down and lacking in energy – and that is just the start of ill health. It is a challenge to alter your way of eating but I honestly believe that so many things in your life can be helped as your health improves, such as your mood, relationships and career. In other words your whole life can be affected in a positive way by this beautiful new healthy you!

If you want to improve your diet and your health, where do you begin? Start by reading the 14 daily menus that follow later in the book. It may seem daunting to try and change your entire diet at once, so why not do it gradually? Choose one day from the 14 options and cook and eat what I suggest for one day. Do that one day a week for one month. See if your health improves or you feel brighter. You may also enjoy the food!

I have deliberately made these menus almost dairy- and totally soya-free. Remember butter is still allowed as it has no milk protein. Be cautious with baked beans of any well-known brand, as they are likely to be soya beans. Always read the label: if the manufacturer does not specify the type of bean used (e.g. haricot), it's likely the product contains soya beans. Whole Earth make organic haricot baked beans. Many cook-in sauces also contain soya too and you will have to be thorough when reading ingredients on labels. Nowadays we also face the issue of genetically modified foods and whether to avoid them or not. Choosing organic food will remove this problem.

I haven't added many nuts to the menus as many people find them hard to digest and we want everything you eat to be easily digestible. The best nuts I can recommend are macadamia nuts; they can be as good for your body as olive oil and eating a few every day will improve your health. I always recommend the soft round lettuce which we call butter lettuce as I find iceberg lettuce hard to digest. For mashing any vegetables please use butter – I think it's better for you than margarine.

These 14 daily menus make a good starting point to improve your diet. It is difficult to plan meals for people without knowing them as individuals, but my suggestions are well balanced and nutritious and a good way for anyone to begin. The foods listed are a minimum amount needed for one day. Please eat and enjoy them. If you are still hungry, eat more of the recommended foods – this is not a restriction diet. These suggestions are simply ways of getting more nutrients into your diet while at the same time eating easier-to-digest food.

Why do I need vitamins?

3

It may be that you do not know anything about vitamins and are unsure of their use and their worth. I personally look at vitamins and minerals as an extra form of food. When trying to explain the benefits of Spirulina I hold up the capsule and say, 'Don't think of this as a vitamin, think of it as the condensed goodness of ten Brussels sprouts.' I'm not exactly a smooth talker, am I? Perhaps this may put some people off! I remember once when my daughter was very young she asked if she had to eat a whole Brussels sprout!

I have often heard people say they know they don't eat enough vegetables. That is why Spirulina is such a fantastic supplement – it supplies vitamins and minerals in a natural form – it's just like eating green vegetables – and can make up for a deficiency in your diet as well as boosting your health.

I recommend many vitamins and minerals in this book and explain why I think they are necessary for a healthy body. I would much prefer it if I could advise you on a good diet which would supply all your nutritional needs. This is impossible for many reasons including over-farmed soil, pollution and your own individual needs and preferences.

How can it be that a lack of vitamins and minerals can make someone overweight? Quite easily. It takes many vitamins and minerals for the body to work properly. All of our organs have different needs and if they don't get what they require to function correctly, your physical health will suffer. You will not digest your food as well as you should, so therefore you will not eliminate properly and that will lead to weight gain. If, for instance, you find you have pain in your joints or perhaps swollen knees or ankles or a pain at the bottom of your back, these can all be signs that you may be lacking calcium and other minerals. Suffering from cramp, perhaps twitching before you fall asleep at night, or having a sluggish system with poor elimination can all be signs that you are lacking magnesium. Our bodies require calcium and magnesium to power our muscles, so a lack of these minerals can cause constipation.

Some people are amazed when they find what a difference a good quality multi-vitamin pill makes to their energy levels. The first thing to consider with a multi-vitamin is can we break it down and get the goodness from it? Some tablets are so tightly compressed they can pass almost unprocessed through the body, and it is common to hear people remark on an unpleasant aftertaste after swallowing vitamin pills. This is because the pills are sitting in the stomach, stubbornly resisting digestion!

I suggest taking digestive enzymes and/or Aloe Vera juice at the same time as your daily multi-vitamin. If you are taking a natural product such as Spirulina then absorption becomes less of an issue. Many of us require large amounts of B complex vitamins and, where our diets do not supply all we need, this deficiency can manifest itself in unexplained anxiety, butterflies or churning in the stomach, shaky hands and broken or sleepless nights.

I always say that B complex vitamins are essential for beauty. They can prevent the signs of ageing by keeping your skin smooth. They encourage hair to thicken and promote its growth, and in large enough quantities can even restore hair colour – I have frequently seen this happen! I have recommended it to many women suffering hair loss due to stress, overwork, grief or illness, to encourage new hair growth. This can take a long time, however, and usually entails an improved diet and large quantities of nutrients for many months. In most cases, though, hair returns with great success and, as you can imagine, the clients feel it is well worth all the effort.

How does all this affect weight loss? As I said earlier, if your organs aren't getting sufficient nutrients to work efficiently, your whole system will be sluggish and naturally this will affect elimination and weight loss. If you are holding on to waste you are holding on to weight.

Most people believe that a good, varied, healthy diet will supply all the vitamins and minerals necessary. I wish this was true. I hear it time and time again when I suggest to someone they may need vitamins and minerals because I believe they are lacking these essential nutrients.

Most people quote the RDA, the Recommended Daily Allowance, and say that they feel they are getting what they need from their food, and wonder why I am suggesting amounts much in excess of this. My reply is that the RDA was established over 30 years ago on a hypothetical healthy person attempting to *maintain* health, who did not have to cope with today's pollution, insecticides, pesticides and over-farmed soil. Most of the people I meet are not in the best of health and may have been living on convenience foods and leading very stressful lives.

The fact is I have seen so many people developing good health, losing weight and brimming with energy after following my advice that I am certain that a sufficient amount of vitamins and minerals can help restore your good health, or even help obtain it for the first time.

It may be of interest at this point to tell you the supplements that I regularly take and also those that feature occasionally:

My regulars: Spirulina
Aloe Vera
calcium, magnesium and zinc
Royal Jelly
betacarotene
vitamin E

Occasionals: ginger
selenium
evening primrose oil
co-enzyme Q10
Milk Thistle
B complex

At the end of this book you'll find information on the products I recommend most frequently.

Should I be concerned about becoming a pill-popper?

4

If you have any worries about taking the vitamins and supplements I'm recommending or suggesting, here are some points you might like to consider.

If you decide you would like to follow my recommendations for a particular symptom and take the supplements, you may feel there are too many pills for you to swallow. Perhaps you could begin by taking the pills just once a day and only take the amount recommended for one mealtime. This means you are only taking a third of the amount I normally suggest. Begin where you feel comfortable and judge for yourself what your body needs. If you improve your diet at the same time, you may need less than the amount suggested. Although I feel I recommend only the minimum amount needed to achieve the maximum benefit, your body may thrive on less – in which case you should reduce your intake.

Let's say you take what I recommend for a particular symptom and you feel better but you don't really like taking these extra supplements. After all, you've read countless times that a good balanced diet should supply all the nutrients necessary for good health. You may be annoyed to read that modern farming techniques mean the land is over-used and the soil depleted, so that the produce grown on it won't sustain good health. Even if you know this is true, somehow you want to fight against taking supplements as you feel it shouldn't be like this. What can you do? My answer is always this: take the supplements. Simply take the supplements. Take them until you feel energetic and achieve the best of health. Once you are in peak health you could use your new strength and lobby the Government to improve farming practices and reduce the use of pesticides, to stop growing genetically modified foods and stop feeding animals with antibiotics and growth hormones. Use your good energy to fight against unhealthy food chain policies.

My advice would be don't fight taking the pills. They are only supplying you with what you need. It should not be a problem to take what's good for your health. Make it a habit. Buy yourself two seven-day pill boxes. Once a week fill one with your breakfast pills and one with lunch. Carry them with you all the time. It is said that it takes 21 days to break a habit and a further 21 days to develop a new one, so if you persevere for three weeks, taking your pills will become like brushing your teeth – just a habit and a very good one.

I've helped so many people regain their health and strength by simply encouraging them to increase their vitamin intake and for some it completely changes their lives and their view of themselves. If you have spent your life being anxious and nervous and unsure of yourself it can be a revelation to discover that this wasn't your true personality, it was just a chemical lack of vitamins. Someone who has suffered this way will soak up vitamins like blotting paper and take them every day for the rest of their life.

A young mother came to me for advice in connection with weight loss. She told me she had been extremely ill after her son's birth seven years previously and how she then had post-natal depression for a whole year. To me the signs were pointing to a lack of all the B vitamins while she was pregnant and throughout all the years afterwards.

Because we had time to discuss her health and symptoms in detail she felt confident about following my recommendation of hourly doses of B complex vitamins for two days, thereafter gradually reducing the dosage until she found the right balance for her. She was so happy to regain her health and confidence – but also extremely angry that she and her son and family had suffered needlessly for seven years. She marched off to ask her doctor why he had never considered that a vitamin deficiency might be behind her problems. I don't know what his reply was, but the doctors I know are under pressure to see a lot of people in a short time and that must sometimes be overwhelming for them. They are trained to save lives and relieve pain and they respond well to symptoms, but when you speak to them of 'feelings' such as anxiety, fearfulness, sadness and unhappiness, they can only listen and suggest a drug – that's what they have been trained to do.

Although it takes years to become a doctor, I believe the time devoted to studying vitamin and mineral deficiencies is very short. You have to be lucky to find a doctor who has a special interest in vitamins, but there are some out there because I've heard of marvellous doctors who sit and listen to their patients and then prescribe vitamins.

During a consultation I have to sit, watch and listen to someone for a long time before I can be sure of what their body may be lacking. I have total faith in the human body to repair and renew itself if we will just listen to it and give it what it needs. Which leads us back to taking your pills. If you have been fortunate enough to discover which vitamins and supplements your body needs to work well, consider yourself fortunate and just take them. How long should you take them? Take them forever – or, to put it another way, take them for as long as you want to be healthy.

I have named and recommended some companies or

brands in this book, but these few are the ones whose products I have personal knowledge of, and I think it's only right that if you are following my advice you should benefit from my hard-earned knowledge.

So to sum up I would recommend:

Take the pills.
Take the pills.
Keep taking the pills.

Do I have to train like an Olympic athlete to lose weight? 5

Often when a woman decides she wants to lose weight she will go about this in two ways – firstly by restricting her intake of food and secondly by starting to exercise more frequently. Well, you will realise by now that I do not believe the first method can really help much and it is my feeling that the second should also be approached with caution.

I can only recommend gentle exercise. I believe that if your body is trying to cope with more weight than it should, strenuous exercise will only put it under more pressure. I believe that making simple exercise, such as walking, gradually become part of your everyday routine is the best way to improve fitness.

Our bodies were made for walking and constant movement, and yet most of us spend our days sitting at a desk or in the car or lounging around watching television. The weather in this country can make it unpleasant for us to spend much time out of doors unless we are very determined. It's also common for work and family commitments to take up most of our time and, although we would like to exercise by running or jogging or working out in the gym, we simply haven't enough time.

I'm always a little worried when someone who is overweight tells me they have begun an exercise programme. I don't want to pour cold water on the idea, because it's probably taken them a long time to get started.

I don't want to discourage them so I usually ask them not to exercise for two weeks until they have lost some weight through changing their eating pattern. Once we have begun the weight loss and they have confidence that the pounds will come off, I then suggest waiting another few weeks before beginning to exercise. Because they are following my advice they feel all right about the delay. My own personal feeling is that I'm not comfortable with any exercise except walking, until some weight is lost.

For me, walking is the best exercise there is and of course if we enjoy the scenery so much the better. Our bodies are more relaxed and comfortable walking than they are at any other time, apart from sleeping. It's best not to carry anything when walking, as the exercise of gently swinging the arms is extremely important and encourages better circulation. The ideal daily walk would be for one hour and although this won't be practical for most people it is something worth aiming for. If this isn't possible, two or three shorter walks would be almost as good. It would always be best to walk in the park, or as far away from main roads as possible, to avoid inhaling traffic fumes.

Most people would accept that exercise is good for their body and for weight loss. When we exercise we encourage our body to work better, we stimulate all our organs, and this in turn helps our body to cleanse and eliminate waste by speeding up our metabolism.

Any weight-reducing diet will be more effective when combined with an element of exercise. This is not to suggest for a moment that you have to take out an annual membership at your local gym or run marathons. I am an advocate of simple exercise such as walking in fresh air.

Exercise can help you lose weight, tone your muscles, and improve your overall well-being. Combined with the right diet, physical activity is the cornerstone of healthy living. Even simple exercise will help you build up strength, endurance and flexibility of your muscles.

So you're looking to lose weight and adopt a healthier lifestyle – how are you going to introduce exercise into this? Start by walking more, and use the stairs rather than lifts and escalators whenever you can. You will feel better for walking to the local shops rather than taking the car. For a moderate exercise programme, walking is the safest and least expensive activity, and you can gradually build this up to longer, brisker walks. Activity breeds activity, and it makes so much sense to live an active life generally. So many people nowadays work at desks or have other sedentary jobs and don't get enough simple exercise. Select activities that you enjoy, and vary them so as to avoid boredom and to involve more muscles. Start gradually and progress at a rate with which you feel comfortable. Apart from walking, any exercise such as swimming, cycling and running will improve your health.

Why do I have sugar cravings? 6

Are mealtimes relaxing and enjoyable for you, or are they fraught with anxiety and guilt? Many of the people I meet feel that food dominates their daily life. They simply can't relax and lead a normal life. They are constantly asking themselves questions: 'What did I eat yesterday? What did I have for breakfast? What can I have for lunch? Should I skip lunch so I can have a meal this evening?'

What a painful way to live. If you become fixated by your food intake, you end up living a life of misery – but it doesn't have to be this way. A truly healthy body will not put on excess weight. That's a strong, powerful message and I believe it to be true. There can be a lot of hurdles to overcome on the road to having a healthy body but I have helped many people to reach that point and you can get there too.

I would describe a yo-yo dieter as someone who feels they have to starve themselves to lose weight. They count the calories and restrict the amount they eat for as long as they can – perhaps a week or ten days – and when their willpower weakens, as it must, and they go back to the way they ate before, the result is that all the lost weight is regained quickly. You are disturbing the chemistry and balance of your body when you yo-yo diet and eventually your digestive system shuts down and you become unable to eliminate the waste from your bowels, meaning the weight will stay on.

You want to be able to eat normally and be slender and yet you just don't know where to begin. First we will talk about your physical body and what you are eating.

Many people have what I call a 'carbohydrate trigger'. This trigger affects your blood-sugar level (BSL) and this in turn affects and controls your appetite. Whether you are satisfied after a meal or still hungry and looking for food depends on your BSL. Let's say your partner enjoys a plate of pasta and salad with you in the evening and afterwards he's content and full – yet one hour after eating, there you are in the kitchen, rummaging around for food. It's clear to me you have a carbohydrate trigger and he doesn't. Poor you, living with a man who can eat anything with no side-effects. Because that's what you are suffering – side-effects from the foods you eat. I hope it makes you feel better to know there is a definite reason for this hunger. It's not just greed or foolish behaviour. So many people have burst into tears with relief when I tell them this. They've felt ashamed and blamed themselves for being weak-willed because they can't stop eating.

The brain requires 30 times more fuel than the rest of the body and it will send you anywhere for sugar until it is satisfied. If that means searching the kitchen or heading out to the shops or the all-night petrol station, then so be it. Remember alcohol turns to sugar so some people bypass the shops and go to the pub or pop open a can instead.

Before I advise you on how to stabilise your blood-sugar level, I'm going to explain what happens and how it affects you.

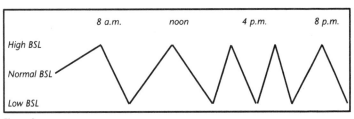

Figure 1

Figure 1 shows how your BSL behaves when you are eating mostly carbohydrates and not enough protein. The level surges up and down, releasing insulin into your bloodstream, then demanding sugar to correct the balance.

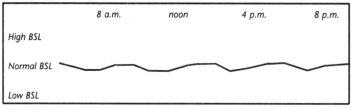

Figure 2

As shown in Figure 2, your BSL remains constant except when you are naturally low on fuel at mealtimes. To achieve this balance you must eat protein at every meal. It is possible to substitute Spirulina for protein at mealtimes.

Someone who can eat what they like and remain slender will be quite likely to have a steady BSL, although whether this is natural to their body or due to their choice of foods is something which we will discuss later.

Let us consider an average day for someone who unknowingly has a carbohydrate trigger. You wake up in the morning and you feel like having just tea and toast. Mid-morning you have coffee and a biscuit. You enjoy a sandwich for lunch and by late afternoon you have another cup of tea or coffee. You get home at five, six or seven and the evening begins. You start to nibble crisps, biscuits or bread while you are preparing the evening meal and by the time the food is ready you are either too tired or full to really enjoy it. You eat it anyway but you are already thinking about what you can have that's sweet afterwards. You spend the rest of the evening in and out of the kitchen looking for something to nibble on. You go to bed feeling bloated, uncomfortable and unhappy. The days you have eaten and felt like this are the ones in which you haven't had enough protein at each meal. It's not enough to have a large steak in the evening and think that's your protein requirement for the day. It can take six hours to digest a steak, so it's likely you will be sleeping before the digestion is complete. Our digestive system closes down while we sleep, so for many people the food can lie in their stomach for days.

If your breakfast and lunch consist mostly of carbohydrates, cereal and toast for example, your BSL will soar quickly. Your body will say, 'That's too much sugar for me to deal with right now.' What will it do? It will flood your system with the most powerful hormone we have, insulin, and this will cause two things to happen. First, the insulin will 'hold' the sugar and control how it's drip-fed into your system. Secondly, it does something amazing as well: it sends a signal that says 'store for later'.

It's possible to eat a plate of plain vegetables with no butter or oil and then a plate of fresh fruit without any yoghurt or ice-cream and yet when these calories are stored for later they are stored as fat. This is all tied in with your BSL. When you have too many carbohydrates without sufficient protein, your BSL rises, insulin is produced and then your body may store these calories for later as fat. We do not want this to happen. We want to keep your BSL as constant as possible so you will use the minimum amount of insulin. As I mentioned above about carbohydrates, your insulin levels can also become trigger-happy and eventually even a small amount of sugar will set off a surge of insulin.

To keep your BSL constant, you have to eat small amounts of protein at each mealtime and preferably this should be spread over five or six small meals every day. Having a routine helps. Eating three balanced meals a day and two small protein-based snacks will really be beneficial for your body. This way of eating helps your BSL in two particular ways. First, your body will adapt to a routine and will help you by releasing extra digestive juices at these pre-arranged times. Secondly, by eating to a plan or time-table, you will usually eat before you are very hungry. If you wait until you are starving it means that your BSL has dipped and it may take hours before you digest the protein and stabilise your BSL again. In the meantime, the trigger and the seesawing of sugar and insulin may begin again.

Most people would list cereals, bread, pasta, rice, beans, potatoes and corn as carbohydrates but may forget that fruit and vegetables are also carbohydrates. Until your BSL has stabilised, you have to be careful to balance your protein and carbohydrate intake at every meal if you can. I advise my clients to do this for three or four months until their health improves. I recommend if you have three or four ounces of protein at a mealtime then you should have no more than eight or ten ounces of carbohydrate – which means your fruit, vegetables and bread and dessert would be included in these eight to ten ounces. Of course, if you have an eight-ounce steak you can have 16 ounces of carbohydrate. These figures are only a guide. Although it may seem quite a rigid way to eat for a while, I don't want to suggest anything that makes life harder for you. My real aim is to make life easier for you.

For anyone who can't eat at a regular time, I would recommend they take two Spirulina capsules three times a day. Many people do not want to eat protein at every meal, or they haven't the time to cook and eat properly. I recommend these clients take Spirulina capsules when they have a protein-free meal, or no meal at all. The vegetable and protein multi-vitamin will help keep your BSL steady and you will not be hungry. You may be able to balance your meals as I suggest only twice a week, and that's fine. Even small changes will help you move in the right direction towards good health.

Now I have shown you how to keep your BSL constant and hunger at bay, what other improvements can you expect? You may lose your feelings of anxiety and your mood swings. You may lose your feelings of constant tiredness and most of your negative thoughts. Can your blood-sugar level really have such a major influence on your body and emotions? Yes, it can and does.

Making a few lifestyle changes

The next step is to show you how to rebuild your health and get back to your good looks and *joie de vivre* (joy of life) and put some spring back into your step. Can we do it? Yes, we can and we will.

Let's begin with an average day in your life. Do you have the bedroom you want and enjoy? How we begin our day and how we live and eat is so important to our health and sense of well-being. Do you allow enough time to enjoy a proper breakfast so you are set up for the day and ready to face the world? If you work in an office and at a VDU screen, do you take all your breaks and lunch away from your desk? Do you try to go for a walk at lunchtime so you can get as much fresh air and sunshine as possible? Do you refuse to spend many working hours in a basement or a room without natural light? If you have a sandwich at lunchtime, do you bring one from home so you know it's fresh and wholesome and not made in a factory two days earlier? Do you try to have a walk before you prepare your evening meal? Do you sit at a dining table and eat without reading or watching the television? Do you enjoy a relaxing bath and a restful night's sleep? Do you treat yourself as well as this? It is not possible for every day to be like this but, in order for you to thrive, you must give yourself this level of care and attention on a regular basis. It's all about taking enough time for yourself.

A good happy way of life will give you a healthy foundation and the magic ingredient of energy or, as I prefer to call it, lifeforce. People used to say 'you are what you eat' but we now know it's 'you are what you digest'. And, remember, if you digest it your body will extract the goodness from it and eliminate the waste and that's exactly what we want it to do. So you are eating good food, digesting it, absorbing the nutrients, eliminating the waste, remaining slim and thriving. What more could we want? That's a pretty good formula for a long and happy life. This is mostly care for your physical body. Emotions and their effect on you will be discussed fully in a later chapter.

If you have been a yo-yo dieter and have read the book so far, you will now know why you were never successful at keeping the weight off, and why you were always fighting hunger. It's all down to your BSL and its fluctuations. It is best not to count calories or restrict your intake of certain foods just because of their fat content. Americans are obsessed with low-fat foods and yet as a nation they are getting fatter and fatter. Fats are essential for health and they do satisfy us so we feel full. If you have been a yo-yo dieter, it will take a great leap of faith to eat as I am recommending. So many people tell me that when they stop starving themselves and follow my advice to eat normal meals, they feel terribly guilty at the start. They are so used to constantly watching calories and fat content that they feel greedy and out of control. But yo-yo dieting doesn't work and you know it. If you follow my advice and give your body a chance to be healthy and fit, the weight will come off naturally and stay off. To keep your BSL constant, I would suggest you take the following supplements:

Two Spirulina capsules before each meal
One 50mg vitamin B complex after each meal
One 200iu vitamin E capsule with evening meal
One 200mg magnesium tablet with evening meal

Is my past making me ill?

Do you believe that your outlook on life can influence your health and weight? It is my experience that a person's outlook is a very powerful factor in weight loss and health improvement. There are many different types of people in this world, but I find it is possible to put people into one of two broad categories – givers and takers. This may take a bit of explaining, but if you read on I think you may recognise some of the things I have noticed, perhaps in yourself or someone close to you.

I have helped many people regain their health and become slim, and it seems as though some of them were just waiting for directions. I advise them which way to go, they ask a few questions, just to be sure they understand me and it's as simple and easy as that. Off they go to success. The younger the client the more likely this is to happen. It's a combination of their attitude and the fact that because they are younger, their bodies respond to treatment and heal much more quickly than an older person's would.

Some people must see an immediate or quick result before they will continue to follow my advice. Quite a few times two sisters have come to me for advice. A month later one of them is still going strong, losing weight and feeling much better, while the other one just will not begin or starts and stops. I've tried to understand why some of us 'fight' success. All we have to do is follow the steps. Obviously I'm not just talking of health and weight loss, but about anything we want to achieve. As the old saying goes, 'You can lead a horse to water, but you can't make it drink.' Why is that so often the case? So many people appear desperate to become slim and yet they spoil their chances. When they consult me they often tell me what they have tried that didn't work, and more or less challenge me to explain why my ideas are bigger, better and faster than what has gone before. They want me to fail with them. Or, to put it another way, they would prefer to remain overweight and prove me wrong rather than lose weight and admit I could be right.

In order to understand and appreciate what the other person is feeling I always try to open myself to them and tune into their feelings. This means I am often successful at understanding them, but it's a different matter entirely trying to influence them. I suppose the easiest people to convince are those who are open to change and willing to try something new. I usually have most success with clients who ask my advice on their health and weight, consider my suggestions and, if I can convince them I know what I am talking about, will give my ideas and recommendations a few weeks' trial. They are not pre-judging me or my advice. They believe I am using my best efforts to help them. They admit they have a problem and want to find a solution. In other words, these people expect life to get better and are cautiously optimistic and willing to accept help.

What if life has always been hard for you and never really gone well? What would you expect from life? More of the same, probably. If you were brought up in an unhappy, troubled home, you may believe that misery is normal and that life is supposed to be like this. If you are put under too much pressure when you are young, if you have to survive in an unhealthy (emotionally or physically) family then I believe this unnatural pressure will push you into an extreme position. In order to survive you will find a way of coping with unacceptable behaviour which can come in many different forms, from control to neglect. If you are the child of an alcoholic parent you may end up being the care-giver, having to protect yourself and also making as few demands as possible. Constantly watching your mother or father to see how they are going to behave today, never being able to relax. Always feeling tense and concentrating on them and what they are doing and not giving enough time and thought to your own needs. You may have been born with a naturally loving and giving nature but this kind of misery in your childhood will force you into an extreme position and you will become a giver.

You may be wondering what this has to do with your health and weight today. Please bear with me and I will show you how your past treatment can influence your life today and a large part of that is what you eat and how you look after yourself.

If you consider that the food we eat turns into energy which gives us lifeforce then it follows that if we don't get the food that's right for us we can't get the life that's right for us. If the obstacles in our life are indigestion, ill health and being overweight, we must clear them from our path. If you were brought up in a large family and you felt you didn't get enough time or attention, you probably still feel that lack. There will be an emptiness inside you and you may always struggle to fill it. Some people are lucky in that they have this kind of childhood, but they marry well. They choose the right partner, someone who will give them and their children a happy home with lots of love and attention, and in this way they get another chance to thrive and develop into a well-rounded, loving and giving human being.

What happens if you are not so lucky and you end up in a relationship with someone from the same kind of family background as yours? Everything will be okay as long as nothing goes wrong. Together you make up a surface relationship with each person looking out for him or herself, except for times when it's mutually beneficial to come together, such as in financial arrangements. If you take as much as you can from everyone around you and never have a sleepless night over the fate of another person then you are definitely a taker.

We now have the two extremes of behaviour of givers and takers. These are the people who are hard to reach or help if they ever become ill or overweight, bulimic or anorexic. If you are a giver and suffer anxiety you may be a yo-yo dieter or bulimic. Anxiety can stop you digesting, so no matter how little you eat it can turn to fat overnight. As I've already said at the beginning of this book, not everyone who is overweight is overeating, they are often just not digesting.

We all know people who, if they eat normally (as in three meals a day), can put on 7lbs over one weekend. That's indigestion; and if every other health concern has been considered and eliminated, the cause can be anxiety. I know some people can be anxious and be skin and bone, but this book is concerned with people who are struggling with weight gain. Someone who is anxious and puts on weight overnight may resort to bulimia since it's bad enough being anxious but anxiety and weight gain is just too much for them to cope with. I helped a lovely woman in her 30s to regain her health. She was extremely insecure about her looks and only felt confident when she was very thin. Her anxiety to be thin made her fearful of food and the little she did eat would lie undigested in her stomach and simply not move. This, of course, led to weight gain. If she had to eat a normal amount at a dinner party or a restaurant, her bathroom scales would show a gain of 3lbs or more the following morning. If she and her husband ate out twice over the course of a weekend, by Monday morning her weight could have increased by 7lbs. She felt that no matter how little she ate she still put on the pounds. She told me that after years of starving herself during the week and eating normally with her husband at the weekend, she simply couldn't take it any more. She had started to eat what she wanted and then throw up after every meal when she had the privacy to do so.

Givers must realise their limits and begin by avoiding situations that are unhealthy for them. Butterflies in the stomach, a churning sensation, fist clenching and a tightness in the jaw are only some of the physical signals your body is sending you, telling you to leave this situation, place or person. I'm not suggesting you have to leave forever, I'm saying leave until you gain sufficient strength and are able to think clearly.

A young mother consulted me about her health. It wasn't too long before it emerged that she was successful in business but was being bullied at home by her husband. As we talked, I also discovered she had such a dislike of smoking she wouldn't allow anyone to smoke in the house including her husband. I pointed out to her that she had decided not to allow smoking but she had decided to allow bullying. If she could be firm about no smoking then she could be firm about expecting good treatment, if she wanted it. That's what I believe a giver must do – decide in advance what they will and will not allow.

Here is one of the stories I use to illustrate this point. You are walking home and a brick hits you on the head. You wake up in hospital and you've lost your memory. A doctor comes in, reassures you that it will return (your memory, not the brick!) in a few days and suggests you go home to recover. If this were to happen to you today, how would your life look to you if you could see it with fresh eyes? Would you be pleased with your home and how welcoming and comfortable it was? Would your husband or partner be pleased to see you and be concerned for your well-being and health and show you this by his attention and care and loving words? Would you get a phone call from your employer telling you to look after yourself but to enjoy a few days' rest, as you deserved it? Would you get calls from friends saying how worried they had been when they heard the news of your accident but telling you they looked forward to seeing you as soon as you felt better? What kind of life are you 'giving' yourself?

I've been consulted by many people who are extremely overweight and regardless of what I advise or suggest, the weight stays on. For some the extra weight gives them a feeling of security, almost as if they had two people to cope with their problems. What about those who must lose weight for an operation or to keep their job and who appear to be following my advice but remain overweight? In the past when I was asked for help I committed myself and agreed to stick with someone until they lost weight. I don't do that any more because I realised my optimism could not overcome their negativity and that I was being drawn into a battle that had nothing to do with me and which I couldn't win. In the past before I learnt this lesson and became embroiled in their problems, they would ask me a question and I would respond with a positive statement. The reply I would usually hear would be 'Do you think so?' and I would be forced to respond positively again. I often felt I was going round in circles. The clincher would be at the end of our long discussion and my pep talk: as they were leaving my consulting room their very last question or complaint would be the very same one that had opened the conversation! I would feel a sweep of exhaustion come over me and realise I had again wasted my time. I would call this type of person a taker, and there are a lot of them out there. I'm still completely open to new people, however, as I always want to be approachable and enjoy new friendships. But I do look out for the 'Do you think so?' reply and in order for me to really learn my lesson, I had to bring it into the open and address it. What I began to do when I met a taker was make it clear I could give advice and recommend products but the problem was theirs. Some pursued me and backed me into a corner until I stood up and said they would have to change their attitude before their life could improve. In other words, they had to think of others. There are still a few takers that slip past my net and then I get that 'Groundhog Day' feeling. That's when it's time to leave. (For anyone who hasn't seen the film *Groundhog Day*, this simply means you keep repeating the same mistake.)

If you are a taker and you want advice on how to improve your life and be healthier and happier, I would say consider yourself as an empty bucket with a hole in it that needs repair. The only way to repair or heal this hole is by caring for others. Give time to someone or something else. Find someone to love and love them for their sake without thought of gain. Altruistic love for others releases the hormone Oxytocin in our brains, making us feel happy and pleased, and the more you set off this hormone the better and stronger the flow. You yourself will gain by giving and become happier and healthier as a result.

What's so good about being a giver? Giving people are supporting and nurturing and give others a chance to grow. They concern themselves with the well-being of others and the world needs them. Einstein once said, 'I don't know anything about you but I do know those of you who give service to others will be the happy ones.' Healthy givers are the people who have plenty for themselves. Plenty of what? I'm not talking about money alone. I had a wonderful aunt who gave to everyone; she had a wonderful husband and he gave to her. A young, happily married couple I once knew with giving natures tried to help everyone who asked them; when she would give more than they could afford, whether that was time or money or both, he would say, 'Let's do what we can for them but we can't take them home and raise them!'

What's wrong with being a giver? Sometimes, someone who keeps giving to one person and who doesn't expect anything back can keep the other person from growing up and maturing. I am not discussing the parent/child relationship here as I do believe that should be a one-way relationship. Let's say a man and woman meet. She is a giver and he is a taker. She gives and doesn't ask for anything back. He takes but feels uncomfortable as on some level this doesn't feel right. He stays out late, doesn't phone and she accepts his behaviour without saying how she feels about it. He stays out late again, and again she doesn't even mention it. He can start to feel almost depressed. What's going on? Does she care or is she just hanging around until she meets someone else? Does she think he's so unattractive that no matter where he goes no one will ever think he's a catch? Or does she think that she's so unattractive that she'll accept his behaviour no matter how bad it is? Before long he begins to wonder if he wants to be with someone who thinks so little of herself. He's off!

Whatever you think of yourself, and however you see yourself, it's only a matter of time before the other person or world sees you the same way whether it's good or bad.

It used to be that single women would claim all the best men were married. What they really wanted was a man who was behaving to the high standards demanded of him by another woman. In their hands, they thought, he would just slip down and behave the worst way they expected. I knew an elderly American man who was a good husband to a demanding and loving wife. When she died he married a woman who had been badly treated and ignored by her own late husband. She didn't have the same expectations as the American's wife and tolerated poor behaviour. Within two years the man behaved in exactly the same way as her first husband simply because he could and she allowed it.

What's good about being a taker? The most obvious thing

that's good for a taker is they keep everything for themselves. Everything good that comes their way stops with
them; nothing gets filtered down to others or given away.
What they can't use immediately will be stored for later.

A woman I knew, who lived in a very small house with
no real display space, inherited a collection of 60 valuable
first-edition plates and 30 crystal vases. She invited her
friends and neighbours round to celebrate her good fortune
and show us the spoils. Out came plate after plate, vase
after vase and we all *oohed* and *aahed* as they were very
beautiful. I was watching her next-door neighbour's
reaction to these prizes and I knew her hopes were high.
She had been a true friend and neighbour to her and was
always helping in so many ways, and every week she
handed in some of her delicious home-baking. She was
extremely house-proud and everything in her home was
spotless and shining. How she would have loved just one of
those crystal vases. She had probably already decided
where it would sit. It wasn't to be. Every beautiful item was
re-wrapped and packed back into its box. No one ever saw
them again. What a wasted opportunity to spread some joy
and pleasure.

If you are a taking person, it's easy to be physically and
mentally strong. If all you have materially you use for
yourself and don't concern yourself with anyone else's
problems or misfortunes, there won't be any leaks of your
energy and you will sleep soundly at night. People will
sense you are not a giver so they won't ask anything of you
and as a result you won't have to use energy saying no. On
top of this natural protection and conservation of energy,
because the world loves balance and opposites often
attract, people with giving natures will want to do things
for you and you will take from them and not reciprocate,
growing stronger all the time. Sounds a good deal being a
taker, doesn't it?

What's wrong with being a taker? Well, there's never any life around takers. Nothing flourishes or grows. It takes a lot of energy and effort to make a difference or change in this world and takers won't get involved. I have always believed that you will receive what you give out, and throughout my life I have seen this time and time again to be the case.

To give is a sign you have faith in this world. You don't believe thieves will come in the night and steal all your treasures. You imagine the world is usually a fair place and that people will help you if they can. Takers don't believe that. They are fearful that they will lose their possessions and, since they have put possessions before people, they will be left with nothing. You'll never hear them say, 'It's only money!'

If you have a taking nature you won't expect anything better from someone else. If you don't have or want to develop a generous nature, you won't value it in anyone. It's said 'a giving hand is a getting hand' and I do know that what you give out you get back, good or bad. If you keep taking from everyone around you, eventually they become exhausted. Love, time or money, whatever you've taken is what they have lost. What happens then?

If you keep taking from someone until they are drained they will become worn out and old before their time. Their health will fail and they will become ill and they will have nothing left to give you and they will be no further use to you. It is important to find a balance in life. In different relationships we take on different roles – sometimes it is important to take what you are offered and other times you yourself must give freely. Problems occur when you live your life at one extreme. Extreme behaviour of any form results in someone suffering, whereas a balanced life with some giving and some taking means that each person will get a chance to thrive.

How can I improve my chances of conceiving?

8

The biggest change for us as women is when we become mothers. I don't believe it matters whether this was a planned and longed-for event or a sudden surprise; in either case it's a shock to your body and your life. Some women find it easy to conceive and others have to wait years. How easy or difficult the birth itself will be is dependent on your health, your emotions and your relationship with your doctor or midwife. Many women enjoy every minute of their pregnancy and really do bloom. Equally, we all know of someone who had to spend nine months resting in bed to have a successful pregnancy. Most women fall between these two groups. They may be happy but they also suffer morning sickness, discomfort and tiredness.

Many couples have come to me for advice on conceiving, some of whom have already suffered miscarriages, and what follows is what I've told them. I will also discuss the common everyday symptoms of pregnancy, and I'll spell out my advice on them. Then, with suggestions from my daughter's recent experience, we'll give you the benefit of our pooled knowledge of how to care for yourself and your baby after the birth. I know that balanced weight and good health go hand in hand and if you can get good advice before, during and after pregnancy, you will not end up overweight or unwell. Tired, yes, but not unhealthy.

Conceiving

You want to have a baby but you are not sure how quickly you will conceive. The best thing you can do is to use this time to prepare, nourish and nurture yourself from this moment on. You can never start preparing too soon. If you want to have a baby in the far-off future, start getting your body ready now. Many of the things you have to consider will apply for the whole of your pregnancy. There are many important things to bear in mind such as what foods to eat and how much rest and sleep to have; the stresses and strains of your working environment and the relationships with your colleagues; and the level of chemical pollutants around you at home and at work. Do you enjoy your home and where you live? What kind of emotional, physical and financial support can you rely on from your husband or partner and close family?

You may have enjoyed a good, happy childhood with loving parents, but your mother or father may not have been interested in cooking or much of a homemaker. Life may have been hectic and mealtimes a bit of a hit or miss with perhaps too many takeaways or convenience meals. I want to show you the best way to begin your pregnancy because 'well begun is half done'.

What to eat

For a healthy mother and beautiful baby I would recommend that around a third of what you eat be protein as in eggs, fish, chicken, lamb and beef. Obviously you should only eat things you enjoy, but if your choice of food is mostly based on habit, or on what your mother served, you may consider trying new things to see if you can develop a taste for them – remember, variety is the spice of life.

The next third of your food intake should be fruit and vegetables, either as part of a meal or during the day and evening. The best time to eat fruit is at the beginning of a meal, but most of us also enjoy it between meals. Fruit is easily digested as it contains its own enzymes, and can move through your digestive system in 20 minutes. The last third of your diet should be cereals, grains and breads, and that's quite easy to do when you consider this includes either cereal or toast at breakfast, a biscuit or scone mid-morning, a sandwich at lunchtime and either rice, pasta or bread with the evening meal, plus the cake or dessert afterwards.

The best foods to eat are those that are organic. Don't make it your life's work to look for them, but buy them if you see them. Have at least one green vegetable a day such as broccoli, Brussels sprouts, cabbage or leeks. The meals listed in the 14 days of menus at the end of the book are a good example of how you should eat. You can, of course, alter and adjust them to suit your own likes and dislikes. It is important for you to know that I don't think it'll do your body any good if you force yourself to eat food you don't like. You won't be able to relax and digest them so you won't get the nutrients from them.

If you find all this advice on food overwhelming, and you are wondering how you could possibly keep it up, just do what you can gradually. Your health will improve with this way of eating and so will your energy levels. You may have been fortunate enough to have been brought up eating this way and you may not have appreciated that this was the reason why you were so healthy. In fact, your diet may now include more convenience foods than your mother ever gave you.

Rest, relaxation and sleep

Are you full of energy, vim and vigour? If you are, it means you are getting enough sleep. Are you sluggish in the morning? Do you find it hard to get up and out of the house? Are you tired after work? If the answer is yes, you need more sleep. How much is enough sleep? You have to find that out for yourself by trial and error. Some people feel great on only six hours' sleep a night and some are grumpy unless they sleep for a minimum of eight hours.

You might say, 'I don't get enough sleep but I spend most of the evening relaxing and watching television so that should help.' This is relaxing but it won't help because looking at the television drains us so quickly of beta-carotene/vitamin A which is, as far as I'm concerned, essential for well-being. So the old wives' tale that television is bad for your eyes is true. To try and give you an idea of its effects, watching television uses up to 50 times the normal amount of betacarotene used in an average day. It's not good news, is it? That's why most people feel lethargic and drowsy after watching television and why, I suppose, most people go straight from the couch to bed despite their previous good intentions of doing the dishes, tidying up or preparing for the morning. The secret would be to do everything important before you settle down in front of the television, as once these rays get you, you may as well say goodnight. If you were brought up by a working mother who would be in and out of the kitchen all night while everyone else watched television and who would be on her second wind as you staggered to bed, at least now you know how she did it. If there are certain programmes you want to watch, why not record them and watch them when it suits you? This way, when the 30-minute video is over, you will probably have fast-forwarded over the commercials and reduced the time to 25 minutes, and you won't be tempted to keep watching. It goes without saying that I am greatly concerned about the health and eye strain of all our children who are being encouraged to work at computer screens at school and at home.

Your working life

Can your job affect your physical health? The answer has to be yes. I'm not talking about emotional stress here, just physical stress. Is there enough natural light in your workplace? Do you work or sit close to a photocopier and its fumes? Worse still, do you work in front of a computer VDU screen for more than one hour a day? There are health and safety guidelines on this and if you work at a screen you should make enquiries either through the Health and Safety Executive, your employer or the computer manufacturers. You have a right to this information and should take steps to protect yourself where possible.

The same advice applies if you have to use a mobile phone for your job. There have been a lot of stories in the press recently of heavy users of mobile phones developing cancers where the phones touched their heads. There was one person recently who tried to make it a requirement for mobile-phone manufacturers to state on their products that 'mobile phones may damage your health'. The Government didn't help him and he lost, but it's only a matter of time before the law is changed and, just like cigarettes, mobile phones have to carry a health warning. (Similarly, the issue of a possible link between miscarriage and working at a VDU is something also to be considered.) To help yourself at the moment you can buy a hands-free attachment, a type of earpiece which keeps the telephone and the radiation which it emits away from your head. One day recently in Glasgow I saw two well-dressed tourists with their lovely young daughter who looked about nine years old. I noticed that she was carrying a mobile phone in a pocket of her dungarees, right beside her heart. I spoke to her parents and told them of my concerns and the stories that were appearing in the papers. They had heard something of this but thought the problem only occurred when you were talking on the telephone. But I believe that the phone can ring and whether you answer it or not, the caller can leave a message; the phone must be switched on and if it's on it will be emitting radiation. This must also be the first time ever that human beings have walked around with strong batteries in their hands or pockets. Reread the instructions that came with your battery charger and you'll be surprised at how cautious the manufacturers are regarding its use.

What can you do if you work for a printer, a paint manufacturer or a firm which produces chemicals or plastics? My advice would be to look for another job. If it's not possible to simply change your job, what else can you do? I would suggest that you work the minimum number of hours you can get away with. Take all your breaks and lunch outside if you can. Spend as much of your free time – before work, after work and at weekends – outdoors. Avoid wearing sunglasses to allow natural sunlight into your eyes.

Thrive at home

It's extremely important for you to make your home as comfortable and relaxing as possible. It's much better to go ahead with changes and alterations before you conceive at a time when you only have yourself and your husband or partner to think about.

I would also recommend that you reduce the number of cleaning materials and polishes in your kitchen or bathroom. Buy, use and store the minimum you can as these all contain chemicals that can adversely affect us. Pot pourri is another chemically laden product, and any soaps, shower gels or bath oils made with synthetic perfumes are best avoided.

What harm can a little synthetic perfume do? Well, you breathe it in and it enters your body and bloodstream. Since it's artificial, it's hard for your body to break it down to eliminate it. In other words, it's a bit like drinking something poisonous. Your body can cope with normal levels of waste and a certain amount of toxins and pollutants, which could be alcohol and traffic fumes. Anything extra, if it happens often, can cause overload. Have you ever been in a newly painted room and got a headache? That's an overload of toxins in your liver. A hangover from drinking too much is also an overload of toxins in the liver.

Your support system

Do you have enough people around you to support and help you? Are you getting the care and attention you need to be healthy and happy? New mothers need a great deal of love and support so that they and their babies can thrive.

This is the time to get your support system in place. Talk about what you want and what's important to you. I don't mean whether you want a boy or girl or what name you will choose, I mean what kind of life you want for your baby and yourself.

No one can ever prepare a new mother for the massive changes that will take place in her life once the baby is born. The birth itself is usually an exhausting experience. It can be traumatic, dramatic and overwhelming, an emotional and physical roller-coaster, and you soon find out that it is only after you have given birth that the real work starts.

There are exceptions to the above. Some babies hardly cry and sleep soundly for long periods. These, though, are few and far between. Most cry regularly and want more stimulation and excitement than simply lying in a crib patiently waiting for the next feed.

Most new mothers get a terrible shock. The baby can be the most beautiful thing they have ever seen, but that doesn't disguise the fact that the first few weeks, months, sometimes years, can seem to a mother like a never-ending marathon with very few rest breaks. Nature intends for us to respond to our baby's needs quickly – that's necessary for survival – so even when common sense would tell you that you simply must sit down and finish your meal (which is important for you and for your baby) you spend the next hour standing rocking your baby in your arm trying to lull it back to sleep. It's natural and right to put your child first, but it is equally important for you to look after yourself too, as you are crucial to your baby and its long-term well-being.

Any mother reading this will know that what I am saying is true. New mothers need a lot of help. Some want assistance and advice with the practicalities such as nappies, breast-feeding in public, and when to start with solid food. Others need help with shopping, cleaning, cooking and tidying up. It can depend so much on your baby and his or her own personality.

If I had to give a piece of advice to prospective mothers I would suggest having enough ready-prepared oven meals as can fit in the freezer (able to be eaten one-handed, i.e. fork only). It would be much better if these could be home-made, either by yourself or someone in your family. If that's not possible, buy a stock of ready-to-cook oven meals. Eat and sleep at every possible opportunity before the birth.

Perhaps I found it harder than most – or it could be that more mothers are ashamed to admit that they found the exhaustion of early motherhood very hard to cope with. When my baby was about six weeks old, I was frequently heard complaining. Why had no one told me how hard this would be? It is still the best thing to happen to me and I was totally content being a mother, but I felt that there must have been a 'hush-hush policy' in operation. I had had no idea that it was going to be so tough. Babies make women out of girls and men out of boys. If you want to do a good job, you have to grow up and sort out your own life so that you are in peak physical and mental condition before you start.

For anyone who wants to conceive, I would recommend certain supplements. Remember you can always start with a lower dose than I suggest and very gradually increase the amounts. Royal Jelly is a complete food for women and it naturally contains vitamin B6. It has been broken down by bees for you so is easy to digest and absorb. A specialist health shop will stock the 500mg capsules (I recommend the 500mg manufactured by Bumbles). Next, take Spirulina as it is a multi-vitamin in a vegetable form and again is a superfood. A superfood contains all the essential nutrients to support life. As an extreme you could live on Spirulina alone. It is 95 per cent digestible and high in iron. The Government now recommends that all mothers-to-be take folic acid. This is one of the B vitamins, so I would advise taking a separate vitamin B complex as well because every time we take an individual B vitamin on its own, we create a need for the others. I would also suggest you take vitamin E as it will help keep your skin supple and because it lubricates your system, prevents varicose veins and haemorrhoids. Last but not least, take vitamin C. I prefer it in a form called Ester C. This is non-acidic vitamin C in a capsule, specially designed not to upset your stomach.

Many brands of Aloe Vera juice have now started to print the warning 'Do not take if pregnant' on the label. This is very disappointing to me as I know of many women who drank Aloe Vera whilst pregnant and breast-feeding. It really seemed to help their digestion and reduce the feeling of nausea. It also cleanses and heals the body.

To help you conceive, I recommend you take:

One 500mg Royal Jelly capsule at breakfast
One 400iu folic acid tablet at lunch after food
One 50mg vitamin B complex capsule at lunch after food
One Spirulina capsule after each meal
One 200iu vitamin E capsule with your evening meal
One 500mg 'Ester' vitamin C capsule after each meal
One 30ml of Aloe Vera juice, before breakfast and dinner

How can I be healthy during and after pregnancy?

9

Congratulations on your good news! You are going to be a mother. I hope you are brimming with health and happiness. The secret for a smooth pregnancy and a good start after the birth is to keep you healthy. The new baby inside you will take all the nutrients it needs from you so we must give you enough goodness for two. In this way, when your baby is born, you will not be nutritionally depleted. There are countless books on pregnancy giving detailed information on all the changes your body goes through during these amazing nine months. It is enough to say here that you must rest at every opportunity. Your body is taking on an immense task and you must help it by conserving your energy whenever you can.

What kind of health problems do pregnant women experience? I usually hear about morning sickness, tiredness, swollen ankles, excess weight, stretch marks, breathlessness, constipation and indigestion, so let's discuss each in depth.

Morning sickness

I've helped a lot of women relieve morning sickness by treating it as indigestion. I've discovered many of my clients who suffered from indigestion before pregnancy go on to have morning sickness during it. I believe that indigestion is caused by a lack or a shortage of digestive juices in a person's digestive system and sometimes that can be caused by tiredness, tension, worry or simply eating foods that are hard to digest.

If you have previously suffered with indigestion and you have it now that you are pregnant, I would suggest that it is a lack of digestive enzymes. If this heartburn is new to you, on the other hand, it may be you have increased your intake of dairy products (for calcium) and you are now having trouble digesting them (I have discussed hard-to-digest foods in Chapter 1). It would be worth reducing the dairy products to see if the heartburn disappears. You can get calcium from other sources, such as fish and green vegetables. In either case, you don't have to worry about taking digestive enzymes as they can only help you. A few with every meal will simply make up for your lack of naturally produced digestive enzymes and will also help you get the goodness from your food. A ginger capsule will warm and stimulate your system and relieve heartburn. Ginger can also relieve travel sickness immediately; in fact, it helps to relieve feelings of nausea in all kinds of situations.

So, for morning sickness, I would recommend that you begin by having smaller meals than before and eating more slowly. The ideal way for you to eat would be six small meals of delicious foods that you enjoy. If you have recently increased your intake of dairy products, try reducing them again for one week and this may help.

To relieve morning sickness I would suggest you take:

30ml of Aloe Vera juice before breakfast and dinner
Two digestive enzymes with each meal
One 500mg Ester vitamin C after breakfast and dinner
One ginger capsule at breakfast and lunch

Tiredness

First we have to establish why you are tired. Is this something new? Were you full of energy before you became
pregnant but have now gradually become tired? If you
followed my advice before you conceived, it's likely that
you simply need more nutrients and perhaps more rest. To
restore your energy, begin by sitting down, putting your
feet up and thinking things through. Are you giving
yourself enough care and attention? You and your baby
must come first. At this moment only you can care for your
baby. After the birth others can help, but at the moment all
the responsibility is yours. Keep thinking.

The practical side of being tired tells me that you are
either not eating enough, not getting enough nutrients or
not getting enough rest, perhaps because you are working
too hard. Perhaps it is a combination of all three. So now
you know what to do. Eat more. Take your vitamins.
Cherish yourself and say no to every unnecessary demand
on your time and energy until you have your strength back.
What concerns me about tiredness is that it might mean the
baby isn't getting enough nutrients, so great care must be
taken.

To give you lots of energy and strength, I recommend
you take:

One 500mg Royal Jelly capsule at breakfast
One 400iu folic acid tablet at lunch after food
One 50mg vitamin B complex capsule at lunch after food
One Spirulina capsule after each meal
One 200iu vitamin E capsule with your evening meal
One 500mg 'Ester' vitamin C capsule after each meal
One 30ml of Aloe Vera juice, before breakfast and dinner

Swollen ankles

You usually hear that swollen ankles are a sign of excess fluid – water retention – but I believe that it's more likely to be a lack of calcium, magnesium and zinc. How can a lack of minerals cause your ankles to swell? I've already explained (in Chapter 1) that I believe we need calcium, magnesium and zinc to run and feed all our organs. We know that your baby has first call on all the nutrients that enter your body and it may be you don't have enough in reserve to satisfy your own bladder and kidneys. Remember these organs are having to work extra hard during pregnancy. If you suffer from cramp, if you twitch before you fall asleep, if you are a restless sleeper, these could be signs of a lack of calcium and magnesium. Make sure you are eating plenty of organic vegetables, dates, sardines and anchovies.

Conserve your energy and rest as much as you can and every time you sit down make sure you put your feet up.

The best supplements to relieve swollen ankles would be:

One 400mg of calcium with breakfast, lunch and dinner
One 200mg of magnesium with breakfast, lunch and dinner
One 15mg of zinc with breakfast, lunch and dinner
One 300ml of Aloe Vera juice with breakfast, lunch and dinner
Two digestive enzymes with each meal

Excess weight

This is a part of pregnancy that some women really dislike. Instead of gaining weight slowly, you pile the pounds on quickly. Is it that you are always hungry and are eating for two? Or are you just eating your usual amount and yet becoming overweight? If you are hungry and enjoy your food and at the same time you are blooming and have no discomfort or digestive problems, then relax, your body knows what it is doing.

If you are always hungry and always eating and yet have discomfort, heartburn and perhaps wind as well, you may be suffering from low blood-sugar levels or indigestion, or perhaps both. How can we tell which it is? You can start by looking closely at the food you are eating. If you eat too many carbohydrates without enough protein, your blood-sugar level will rise and fall, causing you to experience constant hunger. Remember you will now be eating to satisfy a chemical craving for sugar *for your brain* and this may be more than your stomach can cope with.

Let me explain this process again with an example. You eat a meal consisting mostly of rice and vegetables with just a little chicken or other form of protein. Your blood-sugar level rises because of the carbohydrates so your body then releases insulin to balance it and the BSL goes down. It is now too low and your brain craves energy as in blood sugar and sends you searching for something quick and sugary. Your stomach has just started to begin to digest your first meal and then here comes more. Your brain is still 'hungry' and yet your stomach is full. Your brain will win every time. I've heard so many people say, 'I'm so tired of eating and yet I can't stop.'

Begin, if possible, by having five or six small protein meals a day. The hunger may go in a day or so, as soon as your BSL stabilises, but it may just as easily take ten days or more for the discomfort or bloating to leave. It can take this long for the undigested food to leave your stomach and be eliminated to give you a fresh start.

If at the end of two weeks the constant hunger has gone but the discomfort persists, you are suffering from indigestion and a lack of digestive enzymes. (I'm assuming that you are now having small meals spread throughout the day.) Under these circumstances, I would recommend you take:

Two digestive enzymes with every meal or snack
One 50mg B vitamin complex after breakfast and lunch
One 500mg Ester vitamin C capsule after breakfast and lunch
One 30ml of Aloe Vera juice before breakfast, dinner and bed

I've been recommending (and drinking) Aloe Vera juice for many years. I prefer to dilute it with water to make a long drink. 30ml is about an eggcup-full and by pouring this small amount into a cup of water, you will have enough liquid with which to swallow your pills. As I mentioned earlier, I've noticed recently that most Aloe Vera suppliers or distributors are now labelling their products 'Not to be taken if you are pregnant', and I do not know why. One of the large retail chemists started to label the product this way and now the others are following suit. Aloe Vera is simply juice pressed from cactus leaves; it's a completely natural product. My daughter drank Aloe Vera juice before, during and after her pregnancy and she is sure it helped her.

There was a similar problem during the vitamin B6 scare in the mid-1990s when most of the retail chemists removed any B vitamin over a 10mg strength from their shelves. This was during the time the Government was talking about withdrawing any large dose of vitamin B6 from over-the-counter sale. I recently met a woman who had worked for one of these chemists for 15 years and who had taken 50mg of B6 every day for ten years on the advice of her doctor. When B6 tablets were removed from the open shelves and put behind the pharmacy counter, she felt unsure and stopped taking the vitamin. She is now suffering from list-lessness and depression. For this woman, B6 was essential for her moods.

The Government dropped its plans to restrict over-the-counter sales of any strength of vitamin B6; it had been prepared to try and restrict sales of this vitamin based on a telephone survey made in 1986.

Stretch marks

A large percentage of mothers-to-be develop stretch marks. Some have just a few faint marks, but others feel their bodies are scarred forever. We know that stretch marks are caused by, amongst other things, a lack of vitamin E.

There are two ways of getting vitamin E into your body. You can either digest it or rub it on to your skin. When my daughter was pregnant she used both methods. In addition to eating foods rich in vitamin E, she also took a vitamin E supplement regularly. In addition, she used to pop open a vitamin E capsule and add it to a blend of oils. This mixture consisted usually of a base oil such as jojoba, together with some evening primrose oil (again from a capsule), and an essential oil such as either rose, jasmine, sandalwood or frankincense, depending on her mood. She mixed these together once or twice a week and rubbed the oil across her growing bump after a bath. She also had aromatherapy about once every three weeks which helped with skin tone, relaxation and internal cleansing. Although these treatments can be expensive, it is important to be good to yourself during pregnancy, as it is such a special time and one which cannot be replaced. It is also important to acknowledge what an incredible experience it is for your body and reward it for all the extra effort with some pampering!

Stretch marks can be caused by changes in diet as well as by losing or gaining weight rapidly. Many teenagers who become vegetarians develop stretch marks because of the lack of vitamins and minerals normally obtained through meat. Again my own daughter is a good example here. She developed stretch marks after only two months of a vegetarian diet. She reverted to eating meat and began preparing liver and other nutritious food to help her body heal. Although it was a slow, gradual process, the stretch marks did eventually disappear. That experience was one of the reasons she was so vigilant about taking care of her skin during pregnancy.

Breathlessness

If you are short of breath when you climb stairs you may be anaemic. Your face may also appear paler than normal. It may not seem related, but strong healthy blood is needed for a strong healthy baby. Iron-rich blood will carry enough oxygen to your lungs to keep them clear and healthy and remove waste from your body.

Indigestion

Indigestion can be caused by eating the wrong foods for you. It can also be caused by the wrong thoughts, in the form of worry or insecurity.

Your choice of foods, how and where you eat, and how much you enjoy these foods are all indications of how you think of yourself. Let's say you are in a job you love and have high hopes of moving up the ladder within the company. Your boss comes to see you and tells you her house is flooded and uninhabitable, and asks if she can stay with you for a week while repairs are carried out. This way you will have time to plan and discuss the new project in the evenings. Your flat is just round the corner from the office. You can't refuse. Would you be happy to take her home and let her see your life and how you eat and live? Would she be amazed at your well-stocked fridge and cupboards, at the menu planner and 'to do' list beside the phone, the bowls of fresh fruit and all the prepared vegetables and salad ingredients in the chiller? Would she enjoy a bowl of your delicious homemade soup and savour the aroma of freshly ground coffee percolating while you were chopping fresh herbs to add to the omelette you were cooking? Sounds good, doesn't it? To choose the right foods for your body, to eat them in a relaxed manner in a happy, pleasant environment is surely a sign of a successful life. This is how we eat and live when we are on holiday – and what a difference two weeks of care and attention to our needs can make to our health. The difference is usually so marked we can see it in the mirror. It has been said that a sure sign of middle age is when a holiday doesn't help your looks. It can take a lot more than two weeks to make a big difference at that point in life!

To relieve indigestion I suggest you take:

One 30ml of Aloe Vera juice before breakfast, lunch, dinner and bed
Two digestive enzymes with each meal
One 500mg Ester vitamin C after breakfast and lunch

Constipation

Not every mother-to-be will have a problem with constipation but for those who do it is a serious business and deserves consideration. Because the subject is not always discussed, some people believe that if they go to the bathroom twice a week this is normal. It is not. Normal is a bowel movement every day with no discomfort. Anything less is constipation.

There can be so many causes and reasons for a slow-moving system and the more you can find out about what's causing yours, the sooner you can get back to normal. Even if this has been a lifelong problem, it can still be corrected when pregnant and often by a change of diet or attitude or, better still, both.

A lack of fibre in your diet may be your problem. The best way to correct this is to eat two peeled organic apples every day. Foods such as white flour, white sugar, white rice and over-cooked vegetables can make your system sluggish; they require a lot of digestive enzymes to break them down and are best avoided. Too many cups of tea or coffee can slow down your system as well, and alcohol does the same. This is because they affect your blood-sugar level.

Lack of exercise can be a major cause of constipation. A gentle form of exercise perfect for pregnant women is aqua-aerobics. There are classes specifically designed for mothers-to-be. The buoyancy of the water is a wonderful feeling, especially later on in pregnancy when you really are aware of the extra weight you are carrying. There is also a pleasant feeling of camaraderie as all these pregnant women with big flowery swimming costumes lower themselves into the water and loll about on polystyrene floats!

You may have heard it suggested that a person suffering from constipation is someone who can't let go of anything. If you can't let go in a situation it might be that you are fearful of being left with nothing. If you won't throw out or give away your old clothes because you may wear them again, it could mean you don't believe you'll ever get any new ones. So of course you will hang on to what you have. We sometimes keep the wrong friend and family members around us because we believe that having them is better than having no one.

When I speak about the fear of letting go I'm really

talking about stress and anxiety. When you experience any strong emotion, stress or anxiety your body will react as if this is an emergency and will be ready for fight or flight. When this happens, all the energy needed for digestion is immediately diverted to give you the strength to either run like the clappers or stand and fight. This survival instinct is pre-programmed in our brain and, I believe, our tissues, and no matter how we rationalise the situation with our mind that it was only a small argument, incident, concern or worry, our body is ready for a fight to the death.

This is our survival instinct, and to keep it under control we must look at our life, and if necessary analyse why certain people or situations make us nervous and unhappy. Should we avoid them or can we change our attitude to them? Imagine, for example, that your best friend is in an unhappy marriage and won't do anything about it but still wants you to listen while she complains. This is obviously not a healthy position for you to be in. If your heart sinks when she telephones and wants you to listen to another sad instalment, you must protect yourself emotionally because everything that affects you affects your baby physically. There are many things you could say to your friend to make her understand how you feel. Remember this is her problem and not yours, so you don't have to pretend or manufacture problems in your own life to protect yourself from hers. To stop someone else complaining or make them feel better, we can often find ourselves saying things we don't mean or feel. For example, if your friend complains about her husband's timekeeping, you might find yourself agreeing with her and end up saying something disloyal about your own husband or partner or men in general. What's happened, of course, is that you haven't helped or cheered her up, you've only depressed and tired yourself.

How then can you protect yourself? You could come straight out and say you can't see or speak to her as you must put yourself and your baby first. Or you could explain that listening to her problems is making you unhappy and perhaps it would be possible for her not to discuss them with you, but that you would be happy to hear when she had resolved them or had taken some action. Or you could always ask your husband or partner, or mother, or a mutual friend to speak to her and explain how you feel.

To sum up my advice for constipation, be careful of what you put in your mouth. Choose the best foods you can for yourself and enjoy them in happy surroundings. Similarly, be careful of what goes into your ears. Choose happy, positive companions and people who care about you.

The best supplements to relieve constipation would be:

One 30ml of Aloe Vera juice every time you eat
Two digestive enzyme tablets every time you eat
One 200iu vitamin E capsule with your evening meal
One calcium, magnesium and zinc tablet with breakfast, lunch and dinner
One 500mg Ester vitamin C after breakfast and lunch
One milk thistle capsule at breakfast

How can I give my child a head start in life? 10

Having a baby can feel like the best thing in the world. Labour may be long and tiring but the overwhelming joy at your baby's arrival can quickly wipe out any memories of pain and fear. It is not like that for everyone, though. All kinds of new mothers feel all kinds of emotions after the birth of their baby. That is one of the very hard things about becoming a mother: there are so many new – and sometimes overwhelming – feelings to deal with and new situations to cope with. There are so many things to feel unsure about and not know the answer to, but at the same time you are so busy you probably don't even have the time to think things through properly. You just have to do your best at the time and find a happy balance between following your own instincts and taking friendly advice.

It may be that before your baby was born you thought the last thing you would want to do would be to spend a lot of time with other women who were also new mothers. The thought of a coffee morning may have seemed so boring and conventional; yet now you may enjoy and appreciate the great feeling of empathy and understanding to be gained from spending time with other new mums. Some mothers are content to be on their own with the baby for a few months and then they go back to work. Or perhaps women from big families get enough support and reassurance from their relatives and find that they don't need to build up a network of other new mothers. There may be difficulties and disappointments in life but the joy and pleasure of caring for your child can compensate for a lot of these problems.

When your baby is first born it can be a terrible shock – you have to cope with the overwhelming responsibility, the lack of sleep, the change of lifestyle and the pressure on your relationship. Regardless of how much you love your partner there are bound to be some difficulties to sort out. A baby has a huge impact on both parents, but inevitably it is the mother's life that changes more. Your baby will need you first and so everyone else, including your partner, must fall into place after your baby. It really has to be this way, and others must help you do what you want to do and know what is right.

New mothers are bombarded with all kinds of advice and tips from many different sources, and this chapter is another one of them. Although you will know instinctively what is right for you, it can only help to know how some other mothers did things. It can be exhausting thinking about how to deal with all the different dilemmas that come your way as a new mum, but it is also important for you to realise that you are not alone, and that most women feel the same as you do, both physically and mentally, after their child is born.

Breast-feeding

The first issue that mothers face is breast-feeding. Although it is the most natural thing to do, it still can be difficult adjusting to the physical and emotional sensations involved in feeding your baby. One of the best things about breast-feeding is the knowledge that it is right for your baby. It can be very satisfying to know that you really are giving your child what he or she needs by breast-feeding on demand for as long as it is right for you both. Sometimes in the early days when everything seems so erratic and exhausting, one happy feed can be very rewarding and reassuring, reminding you that you are managing as a mother and that you are doing the job which nature intended.

Different mothers have different feelings about breast-feeding. It is a personal thing that affects us all differently. Many find it a source of comfort and pride, although physically very draining.

Indigestion

Apart from the emotional side of caring for your baby, we also have to consider his or her physical needs. If you have read the chapter on conception you will be aware of the requirements of your own digestive system. But what of your baby's system? They can have indigestion too. They can't tell us where they feel pain, they can only cry and show us their symptoms of discomfort. When I see a baby with a constantly running nose or one who dribbles all the time, I would normally assume the baby is not digesting his or her food properly.

I look on colic as a form of indigestion too and any baby pulling his legs up as a result of wind I would consider to be suffering from indigestion. Constipation or diarrhoea to me also indicates indigestion. I believe that diarrhoea is just nature's way of eliminating constipation. I may ask a mother if her baby has constipation or any difficulty with bowel movements. Some agree that the baby has to strain to have a bowel movement or what he or she does pass is hard and looks like pellets. This is a sure sign the food has been in the system too long. A mother may say her baby has the opposite of constipation – i.e. diarrhoea – but I believe they are one and the same problem. If a baby cannot digest its

90

food, it will stay too long in the stomach and then remain too long in the bowel. If food moves at a normal rate along the colon or bowel, all the essential nutrients will be extracted from it and the waste will be eliminated as a bowel movement. If the food enters the colon or bowel in an undigested form, your system may not be able to move the food in your bowel. It will become dry and hard as it sits there – and your body does not want this to happen. As I keep saying, the body is so perfect it never makes a mistake. To get this waste moving, your body will draw moisture from the rest of your colon and bowel and this extra liquid and undigested food will be passed as diarrhoea. That leaves us with at least two problems. First, we haven't obtained all the necessary nutrients from our food, and second we've robbed the rest of our colon of essential moisture which will be needed when we next eliminate.

Cold fingers and toes and perhaps a slight damp feeling in their hands can be further signs that a child is suffering from indigestion. Babies with cold fingers and toes may not want to sleep in their cots, but prefer to be in bed beside you for warmth (not to mention the simple pleasure of being close to their mother).

When I suggest to a woman who is giving her baby formula milk that the child may not be digesting the cow's milk protein, I am often told that the baby is fine during the day and only cries at night. There can be two reasons for this. Suppose I offered you three bars of chocolate at breakfast. You might enjoy them. If I offered you three more at lunch, you might still eat them, but if I gave you a further three at dinnertime, your stomach would feel queasy or you might even be sick. That's what can happen to a baby who is fed something that he can't digest. He takes his first bottle of the day because he's hungry and thirsty. He may show signs of discomfort or bring up a little curdled milk; however, he is warm and perhaps enjoys his bath and he also has your warmth and company. After the second bottle he may sleep, and again because he is warm he will digest some of the milk while he sleeps. The contents of his bottles will lie in his stomach and by evening or when he goes to bed his discomfort and pain will be at its strongest.

Suppose your baby shows signs of discomfort and yet you are breast-feeding. This could perhaps mean that he cannot digest the cow's milk or soya products you yourself are eating and which will be present in your breast milk.

It's a big step for any mother to remove cow's milk from her baby's diet. She has been told milk is essential for strong teeth and bones. To my mind, though, the only one who gets calcium from cow's milk is a calf. It follows that if your baby is not digesting – i.e. breaking down – cow's milk then he will not get any calcium from it. My first suggestion would be to use goat's milk for you and your baby. There is a very good goat's milk formula for babies called Nanny's. Most health-food shops either stock it or can order it from a wholesaler. This product is well known and some parents end up simply preferring goat's milk to cow's. Goats are not subject to the commercial farming that cows endure. They have a more 'free-range' life and will not have been fed with so many hormones. So think of changing from cow's to goat's milk as something positive you are doing for your baby's health.

So many women have told me that when they removed cow's milk products from their baby's diet the difference was so noticeable that they felt as if they had a different baby! The child's colour improved and there was no need for them to wear a bib all day as the runny noses and drooling stopped within 48 hours of the change of milk. Instead, they had no more colic, no wind and a full nappy once or twice a day, as it should be. The mothers found they had a more contented baby, enjoying his feeds and sleeping soundly.

If you are breast-feeding and you change to eating goat's milk products and eliminate all soya products from your diet and yet your baby is still in discomfort, what else can you do? Cut out the goat's milk products: one person in a hundred can't digest even them, and that person could be you. You can get all the calcium you need from organic vegetables, dates and sardines and many other sources.

But what if your baby is being bottle-fed? I would recommend stopping all goat's milk for 24 hours and during this time give the child a drink called Rice Dream. It's a watery-looking milk made from organically grown rice and it tastes sweet although it contains no sugar. It's available from health-food shops and good delicatessens. I am not suggesting that you substitute Rice Dream for baby formula or milk, I'm only recommending you do this for 24 hours to give your child's system a chance to be milk-free. If during this time your baby is free from colic, wind or drooling, it may be a sign that he cannot digest any animal's milk. So what can you do? First of all, relax. It's more common than you think. The one thing I would avoid is a soya or vegetable baby formula because if your baby can't digest cow's or goat's milk, these substitutes are likely to be even harder to break down.

One of my clients has three sons and none of them can tolerate animal or soya milk. She herself was fed on puréed beef and chicken when she was a baby and she did the same for her family as that was all that was available at that time. Nowadays I would suggest feeding a baby puréed vegetables with some Spirulina powder added to it. Spirulina, as I've said before, is a protein and vegetable form of multi-vitamin. The protein is 95 per cent digestible and it's a superfood. It's green and may look strange but it's tasteless and yet so nutritious. Open up one Spirulina capsule and stir or whip the powder into the purée once a day. When the baby is older the powder from one capsule can be added to their fresh juice at breakfast. I have clients throughout Great Britain whose children swear by Spirulina. One of my favourite clients was a nine-year-old who always said, 'Spirulina does the trick,' and he was right.

Skin problems

If your baby ever has dry skin or small raised patches or bumps on his body, nappy rash or red, rough areas on his face or arms, this can be a sign of milk intolerance or a lack of essential fatty acids. If the digestion and discomfort problem has disappeared but the child's skin looks and feels dry in patches, I suggest you add evening primrose oil, which contains essential fatty acids, to his diet. The best and simplest way to give your baby the evening primrose oil is to buy a box of the 1000mg capsules. Leave the lid off the box so the capsules will soften and be easier to cut. After his bath and when he's dry, take one of the large capsules and cut into it at the top, keeping it upright so the oil stays in it. Pour the oil into the palm of your hand and massage your baby with it. Put some of the oil on the child's forehead, cheeks and chin and even into his mouth.

A woman brought her 18-month-old boy to me for advice about eczema. He was completely covered in bandages, with only his face and hands open to the air. These were badly cracked and so painful to look at. His mother said he screamed when she bathed him. I began by cutting open an evening primrose oil capsule and started to gently pat his palms and fingers with it. He let me do this. I then patted a little of the oil on his face and then put some oil on his mother's fingers and she put her fingers to his lips and he licked them. I then opened more capsules and she squeezed them directly into his mouth so that very little of the oil was lost. It was unbelievable to watch because when he first tasted the evening primrose oil, he loved it and kept shouting, 'Again!' We fed him at least 12 of the 1000mg capsules and he smacked his lips and shouted, 'Again!' after every one of them. I gave this young mother as much help and encouragement as I could and I would like to think that she continued with the advice that I gave her.

I advise every mother I meet to give her baby evening primrose oil and also to take it herself, preferably a minimum of 3000mg a day with her evening meal. May I boast at this point that my grandson has perfect skin? My daughter and I are certain that evening primrose oil plays a big part in this.

Personally, I get indigestion if I eat any microwaved food. Have you ever microwaved a bread roll, not eaten it straight away, and when you pick it up ten minutes later it's as hard as a rock? That worries me. I wouldn't take any chances with your baby's food or bottles. Don't use a microwave for anyone you love.

To me, this chapter is the most important in the book. I'm a happy mother and a doting grandmother, and my heart goes out to every young mother and new baby I see. I have learned so much about health and what the body needs to thrive that I feel I must advise and help wherever I can. There are so many pollution problems affecting each and every one of us that bringing up a healthy baby is a harder task nowadays for any mother than it was when my daughter was born. I am more aware of this today because I very recently helped my daughter care for her baby for the first few months of his life. I was so concerned to read that some carrots have 22 times the permitted level of pesticides that we had to buy organic fruits and vegetables to give him a healthy start in life. Because I am so aware of all the many issues relating to good health today, I am overly anxious about my grandson's diet. As a result, my daughter sometimes finds it hard to keep up the level of optimum nutrition all the time.

I hope that you will use my suggestions for your baby's well-being and that you will be rewarded with better health for both of you and a happy time.

How can I feel well during my menstrual period?

11

I meet a lot of young women who suffer from pre-menstrual tension (PMT) every month, sometimes for as much as two weeks in every month. They may experience a lot of unpleasant symptoms such as bloating, tender breasts, constipation, mood swings and especially cold hands and feet. Some women have told me they need to have two different wardrobes as their shape and weight can change so much during this time.

If you suffer in this way, I recommend you try following my advice on cleansing and eliminating. Use the suggestions for a cleansing diet given in Chapter 1 – prepare nutritious, home-cooked meals rather than convenience foods, and eat them while seated at the table. Remember to chew well. Cut down on or eliminate hard-to-digest foods, and drink as little tea and coffee as possible during this time.

A lot of the women I know who suffer from PMT are, in my opinion, anxious and nervous during the rest of the month as well. Your body needs a lot more B vitamins during your menstrual period than normal and many women find just one 50mg B6 vitamin is enough to remove any feelings of anxiety. If you would describe yourself as an anxious person who is sometimes unsure of herself, I would recommend you start taking royal jelly every morning. Royal jelly is the most amazing food for women, and because it has already been digested for us by bees we can

97

absorb it into our systems almost instantly. It seems to satisfy and feed us almost in an emotional way. I think of it as a superfood.

In my experience, evening primrose oil helps us in much the same way, as it seems to calm the body and the nerves. I believe it can soak up the ill effects of any stress hormones we may release when we are anxious. I recommend you take at least 3000mg every day. Try cutting the capsules open, then swallow the oil and discard the shells.

Why do so many women experience bloating just before their menstrual period? I believe the ones who suffer this discomfort are usually experiencing constipation for most of the month. If your system is slow-moving – which means the food you eat is not always properly digested and not being eliminated fast enough – then your bowels will not be emptying properly every day. Your womb may swell slightly during your menstrual cycle as a result of the extra hormones you are producing and it may press on your colon and cause your bowels to empty quickly. This is almost a spring clean for your system and usually once this happens the swollen stomach and discomfort disappears. It would be much better, of course, to have your system clear itself every day naturally.

It may be that a lack of calcium and magnesium is causing the bloating and constipation, and if you crave chocolate just before your period you may be really craving the magnesium that chocolate contains.

So, remember, to relieve PMT have five or six small meals a day, avoid hard-to-digest foods and eating late at night. Make sure you have enough rest and plenty of enjoyment.

To relieve pre-menstrual tension, take these supplements for the whole month:

One 500mg royal jelly capsule at breakfast
30ml Aloe Vera juice before every meal and at bed
Two digestive enzymes every time you eat
One 50mg B complex capsule after every meal
One Spirulina capsule after every meal
One calcium, magnesium and zinc tablet at dinner and at bedtime
Three 1000mg evening primrose oil capsules with dinner

If you are taking the birth-control pill you may not suffer PMT but may, on the other hand, feel bloated and put on weight. A lot of young women I have met stopped taking the pill because they kept gaining weight month after month. It wasn't the usual kind of weight increase – more a thickening around the waist and a puffiness in the face, meaning they ended up looking more unhealthy than over-weight. These changes can happen so gradually and take place over such a long period of time that sometimes it is not until you look at an old photograph of yourself or meet someone you've not seen for years that you realise how much your appearance has changed.

Remember that when you take the birth-control pill you are taking extra hormones into your body and that eventually these hormones must be broken down and eliminated. This is not always easy to do. As I discuss in Chapter 12, Gamma Linolenic Acid (GLA) is essential for breaking down, utilising and eliminating cholesterol and saturated fats from the body. I believe we may need extra GLA (as in essential fatty acids) to eliminate these artificial hormones. Evening primrose oil supplies GLA and that is why many women on the pill feel their health improves when they take 3000mg of EPO with their evening meal. Because EPO helps your body eliminate any waste through the bowels, you will be rewarded with softer, smoother skin, clearer eyes and, of course, weight loss.

12

Is there really such a thing as a mid-life crisis?

Have you had time for yours yet? What is it? How will you recognise it?

It's the day you don't recognise the reflection in the mirror. The sudden dawning. What happened? Where did your youth go? Perhaps we judge the state of our own youthfulness by looking at our partner. That would explain why some middle-aged people embark on relationships with much younger partners. Is it what you see in the mirror that prompts the crisis? Or have the crises you've lived through made the reflection what it is? If you feel a facelift would change your life, it's the reflection that's the main problem. That's why a new hairdo and a new outfit can make such a difference. You'll look more like your 'old' self or your 'newer' (younger!) self, the one that you expected to see in the mirror.

Will improving your health make you look and act younger? Yes, it will – and one of my clients proves this to me every time I see her. We met five years ago when she was concerned about her health. One of my recommendations to her was to take Spirulina, that vegetable form of multi-vitamin, every day. I suggested three capsules a day but she thought I'd said three capsules *after each meal*. She bought a large supply of the Spirulina and didn't visit me for two months. When she came back I hardly recognised her, she was so full of health and vitality and youth. She now looks about twenty years younger than her age. Whenever I see her it reminds me of how fantastic Spirulina is and I always rush to take a handful of capsules! Her aim was to regain her health to enjoy her life and she now has her health *and* beauty.

Rejuvenation is the main reason I became interested in alternative health. I went to live in California when I was 18 and I worked with a woman who was in her 60s but who looked much younger than her years. I watched what she did, what she ate and where she shopped. I decided to follow her example. At that time in California there was a chain of health-food shops called In the Pink – and that's how I feel today thanks to her and her lifestyle.

Can you be happy without being healthy? Let's just say it's easier to be happy when you are healthy. Being healthy gives you confidence and enough energy to try new interests. Being healthy gives you the strength to work hard and yet still have the energy to socialise. When you're healthy you can cope with the daily mishaps and problems of life and just see them as they are without exaggerating their size or importance. If you know someone – and we all do – who makes a mountain out of a molehill, it's easier to sympathise with them if you realise that it's a lack of strength that's causing them to behave that way. It's the equivalent of a cavalry charge. They haven't the energy or strength just to do the task, so they have to run about shouting and increasing the frenzy until they have worked up enough steam to charge up the mountain – because it does feel like a mountain to them.

Sometimes, watching your husband or partner going through a mid-life crisis of his own is enough to bring yours on. Fear is contagious and fear is what I believe we are experiencing at this time. What are we afraid of? Are we scared of feeling unloved, unattractive, unwanted and not appreciated whether at home or at work? Is it fear of financial responsibilities, or fear of running out of time, being left unable to achieve any of the things we want? Are you fearful of the future because you don't like what you see on the horizon?

Many women get a new lease of life when their children leave home, because for the first time in many years they can concentrate all their energy on themselves and their own health. I know that this often comes around the same time as the menopause, and it can be a combination of new signals and changes from your body which makes you nurture yourself and pay more attention to your physical body's needs. When you do this, the increased energy and lifeforce make you look around and say, what's next? What can I do now? Some women wonder why they didn't make such changes earlier, but it's quite likely that all their energy was being poured into their children and family life and that was all they could manage to do at that time.

Most of us don't have the time or the energy to think through or even be aware of all our fears; we only recognise the feelings as anxiety and stress. To relieve these emotions we may drink more, work more or eat more, or look for a new romance. It can take a major event such as an accident, redundancy, illness or even death before we stop and think of where we are in our lives and how we feel about that.

Let's say you are rubbing along well enough with your husband or partner. You live where you do because of his job and that has always influenced your own employment opportunities. He decides he wants to take early retirement and suggests you both leave the city and move into the countryside. You are only now moving up the career ladder yourself, however, or perhaps you're just doing a job you enjoy. This move would mean you would have to stop working. Your husband can't see anything wrong with that because he has always been the main breadwinner. He doesn't understand why you won't just jump in with him and relax in this new life. As you watch him make light of this move, you realise that the two of you have never sat down and discussed the future together. You were too busy as a wife and mother to plan ahead. Most couples work out a balance, but instead of these changes and plans being discussed and anticipated in a positive way, they can be the cause of friction and hard feelings if one partner just suddenly springs their 'desires' on the other. Of course, if your husband has heard you say you are tired of all this work, he may be hurt and disappointed that you are not thrilled and grateful for his offer to take you away from it.

It can be difficult to accept that we are partly responsible for this confusion and all these crossed signals. Many people just don't say what they want. Sometimes if we are so busy just coping with the present we don't take the time to stop and think about what we actually want out of life. If we are not sure ourselves then how can we expect someone else to predict it?

To help with rejuvenation, I recommend you take:

One Spirulina capsule after each meal
One 50mg B complex after each meal
One 500mg vitamin C after each meal
One 200iu of vitamin E with evening meal
One 15mg of betacarotene with evening meal
One multi-mineral with evening meal
One 30mg of Aloe Vera with evening meal to help digestion
Two digestive enzymes with each meal

Remember that taking these capsules even once a day with your evening meal will help you regain your glow.

Is it possible to have a symptom-free menopause?

13

Being on hormone replacement therapy (HRT) can make you overweight. The doctors say that it can't, but my clients say it does. So many women tell me they never had a weight problem until they started HRT. Their lifestyles and eating habits have remained the same as they were before the treatment started, and yet the weight somehow keeps increasing. It's very demoralising for them to be told by their doctors that it's just their age, or to be given a calorie-counting diet sheet, which they know won't help them but which implies they are overeating.

This is an important topic and anyone considering HRT will have to do a lot more of their own research. It's a big decision and it deserves in-depth consideration. I myself would never have HRT. Then again, I would never agree to have my tonsils or my gall-bladder removed, as this is totally against everything I believe about the human body being a perfectly balanced, self-regulating organism which knows how to correct itself. The whole point of this book is to give advice so that you can listen to what your body is telling you and help it to heal itself. I don't want you to have parts of your body removed if there are other ways of dealing with your symptoms. It is the same with hormone therapy: I really feel that HRT alters a crucial part of your system and actually interferes with your body's natural adjustment to life. Yes, you may feel unwell as you reach the menopause and you may be lacking a variety of things such as nutrients, care, love and satisfaction, but these can all be dealt with directly rather than covering them up and blaming these deficiencies on 'the change'. Otherwise you are only masking problems which will resurface eventually.

I'm going to do my best to explain to you what I think HRT does for our bodies. The question I hear often is 'Is there a natural alternative to HRT?' and the only answer I want to give is 'Yes, and it's called good health'. Most doctors are overworked and too busy to have enough time with each patient and I know they try and give as much information on HRT as they have. However, HRT is really quite new and we are still learning about potential side-effects.

HRT floods our system with hormones, fools the body into believing we are younger and encourages it to keep doing the 'youthful' chemical reactions it has always done. One of these hormonal actions is to coat our bones with a form of sheath so the bones can't leak calcium and cause or encourage osteoporosis. As you read on, you'll see I don't agree that this is always such a good thing – HRT may prevent your bones leaking precious materials, but it could be that your body knows best, that it's what your body is designed to do. That's what I believe – read on and see if you agree with me. Remember HRT is an artificial hormone and no one really knows the correct or safe dose. It might be that less is best. Obviously my advice may be of more help to someone who hasn't begun to have HRT although my health advice is for all women. Please continue having your HRT and make the health changes as you can.

The health changes I recommend can help you be healthy or healthier than you presently feel. Some women will only be able to have HRT for ten years because of their family health background, the reason being the increased likelihood of a blood clot developing. If there comes a time when you have to stop having HRT then hopefully having read this book and followed some of my general advice, your overall health will have improved. You will feel better physically than you previously did and your body should cope with the hormone-level changes more easily.

Remember it's my intention to show you how to be slim for life, and that goes hand in hand with good health. In my opinion, every time we take a foreign substance into our bodies, in this case HRT, there will always be side-effects, because your body must process this substance and eliminate it and that involves all your organs and obviously includes your liver and kidneys.

As a woman grows older she runs out of reproductive hormones. This is natural and what nature intended. If she has very good health and a happy enjoyable life and is in a secure, loving relationship, she may not be aware of the reduction of these reproduction hormones because the other 'happy person' hormones, ones that affect our emotions, will continue to flood her tissues and life will go on as it did. (We really do release a 'happy hormone' – it's called Oxytocin. See Chapter 7 for more information about it.) Her ageing process will continue and she may notice more lines and grey hair, but it will seem to be as gradual as before the menopause.

If for ten years before the onset of the menopause life was hard for you – too many problems and worries and not enough time spent looking after your physical body – it's likely you will feel physically and emotionally worn out before the menopause begins. Or let's say you're in your early 40s and you've experienced the usual ups and downs of life, you are working full time and running a house. Perhaps your husband or partner is under stress at work and unable to give you the support you need. Your children may be teenagers or young adults, unsettled and unsure of their future regarding their careers or relationships, and may need your care and guidance. You might have elderly or sick parents who now need more of your help and time than ever. These problems or pressures are experienced by every family; we all have to cope with them and keep going. If you have managed to keep yourself in one piece until now it's maybe because you started out with a strong constitution. You may have come from a family of healthy people. You've realised over the years that you need more rests, more breaks and more holidays – in other words, more care and attention – but there is never enough time or money left over that you can use for yourself. As you enter your mid- or late 40s and head towards the menopause, how your body reacts to the imminent changes is, I believe, totally dependent on your physical and mental health at this time.

What are the symptoms we usually associate with the menopause? Weight gain, hot flushes, tender breasts, sore joints, dry skin, shadows round the eyes, tiredness, feeling sluggish and slow and erratic moods or emotions are all on the menu. Not a very enticing list, is it? But before you rush to the doctor for an HRT prescription, could anything else be causing these symptoms?

Weight gain

I've previously explained what can cause weight gain and how you can remedy this. The major points to consider are:

- the body not cleansing
- poor digestion
- a lack of vitamins and minerals
- eating hard-to-digest foods
- a lack of simple exercise

So I would suggest you consider a detox programme, eating

three simple meals a day, varying your diet and not overeating when you are too tired and stressed to enjoy your food.

Hot flushes

I always look on hot flushes as your body trying, and not succeeding, to eliminate waste. To me, it is a sign that your body is trying to clear toxins by perspiring, so, again, detoxing will help here. Help yourself by drinking Aloe Vera as though it were water. The waste that should be eliminated through your digestive system is trying to escape through the biggest organ you have, your skin. Wearing only natural fibres such as cotton, silk, linen and soft wool will help absorb the waste your skin is emitting, whereas man-made materials will prevent your skin breathing and make the problem worse. Sometimes something as straightforward as your bed linen could be aggravating the situation. It may be that your polyester duvet is adding to your nightly discomfort. Cotton sheets with wool blankets on top might be a better solution and obviously cotton nightclothes will keep your skin cool. I always check clothes labels thoroughly. My body is very sensitive and I can only wear natural fibres – even lycra in tights makes me feel like my legs are wrapped in cling-film!

Tender breasts

I believe this is also a side-effect of poor elimination, and I am sure this is waste being stored in the soft tissue of the breasts. This sounds awful, doesn't it? One of my clients couldn't allow her young son to cuddle her without her saying, 'Be careful, be careful. Not too tight!' After detoxing and two months of drinking lots of Aloe Vera the problem disappeared – and this was something that had been troubling her for ten years. To relieve hot flushes and tender breasts, I recommend you take:

One 30ml of Aloe Vera with every meal and at bedtime
Two digestive enzymes with each meal and snack
One Spirulina capsule after each meal
One 50mg vitamin B complex capsule after each meal
One 500mg vitamin C capsule after each meal
One St John's Wort capsule at breakfast

Sore joints

Sore joints can be caused by a deficiency of calcium and magnesium. A lack of these minerals can also cause your wrists, hands, knees and ankles to swell. I believe the body needs calcium and magnesium as a car needs petrol. All your organs require these essential minerals in order to be healthy. Your heart, lungs, liver, spleen, bowels and kidneys are all using the calcium and magnesium you have in your body. To keep your organs in proper working order, your body will take the calcium it needs from your bones and joints. It follows that if your joints are sore, stiff or swollen, I am certain you are lacking calcium, magnesium and zinc. Why am I so sure? I've seen so many people recover from arthritic problems by taking a good-quality calcium, magnesium and zinc supplement.

To ease pain in your joints I recommend you take:

One 30ml of Aloe Vera with each meal and at bedtime
One calcium, magnesium and zinc tablet after each meal
Two digestive enzymes with each meal
One 200mg magnesium tablet at bedtime

Pain that has sometimes been suffered for many years has disappeared within weeks. If they can afford it, I always recommend that my clients take Aloe Vera and digestive enzymes along with these minerals to aid absorption and therefore increase nutritional benefit. But even simply taking calcium, magnesium and zinc on their own has tremendous effects.

Dry skin

Skin that's dry with rough patches and that sometimes looks red and blotchy can have many underlying causes. First, it can be faulty elimination, and following a detox programme will help here. It could be down to poor digestion which would mean you are not extracting the nutrients from your food. It can also be a lack of oils in your diet. There has been so much publicity about the amount of fat in our food that many people try to avoid fats and oils, thinking these are bad for them. Oils are essential for good health and I make sure I have two tablespoons of olive oil every day, either cooking my food in it or using it in salads. Stress and anxiety can also make your skin dry, as can working with or near chemicals or fumes. One of my clients has a small printing business and I can always tell by his skin condition how busy the firm is.

I would also recommend you take a strong B vitamin complex, at least 50mg of all the B vitamins twice a day. With your evening meal, take evening primrose oil and at the same time some magnesium, as it takes this mineral and B6 to convert the oil into Gamma Linolenic Acid. GLA is an essential fatty acid and it is necessary if the body is successfully to utilise and eliminate cholesterol and saturated fat. I always advise my clients to bite into the evening primrose oil capsules and swallow the oil – it's almost tasteless – and spit out the capsule shell. Have a piece of bread and butter at the same time if it helps the oil go down. This way you are not wasting those precious digestive juices on a gelatine capsule which has no nutritional benefit in itself. We want to save those juices for the food you eat.

For soft, smooth, healthy skin I recommend you take:

One 50mg of B complex vitamins after each meal
One 500mg vitamin C capsule after each meal
One 200iu vitamin E capsule with your evening meal
One 15mg betacarotene capsule with your evening meal
One 200mg magnesium tablet with your evening meal
Three 1000mg evening primrose oil capsules with your evening meal

Shadows round the eyes

When I see someone with dark shadows round their eyes, I think two things are usually to blame – either anaemia (iron deficiency) or a lack of betacarotene/ vitamin A. How can you decide whether you are anaemic or lacking betacarotene? If you are always tired, have heavy menstrual bleeding and feel breathless going up stairs, I would say it's anaemia. If you spend too much time indoors and therefore don't get enough daylight or sunlight, and you work at a VDU screen or watch a lot of television, I would predict that you are lacking betacarotene. I usually ask my clients if their eyes appear smaller than they used to, and if they say 'yes' then I know it's definitely a lack of betacarotene.

Scientists believe betacarotene is changed into vitamin A, or, perhaps I should say, can be used as vitamin A in the body; however, I have found that many of my clients don't seem to be able to convert readily. You have to be cautious when taking vitamin A as any excess will be stored in the liver. Betacarotene, on the other hand, will be stored under the skin, and if you take more than your body needs, the worst outcome is that you'll get a lovely carroty glow! It can't harm you, and will fade within a day or so if you reduce the dose. Betacarotene is an anti-oxidant and helps kill free radical cells when taken with other anti-oxidant vitamins. These free radicals can cause cancer so, to invert what Americans always say, 'better red than dead'.

A woman came to see me about losing weight. She also had huge dark circles round her eyes. Her eyes were so small and tight-looking that she almost had to tip her head back to look at me. We started on the weight loss programme and for her that included lots of vitamins, minerals and large doses of betacarotene. We began with two 15mg capsules a day but she had to work up to eight capsules a day before we saw an improvement in her eyes. She kept up this high dosage along with her other supplements and at the end of four months the excess weight was gone and, unbelievably, the dark circles had totally disappeared and her eyes were wide open and round like a baby's. She looked twenty years younger and stunning with those beautiful wide eyes.

It's possible to get betacarotene from natural sources such as organic carrots, peaches, apricots, mangos, yellow peppers and any other yellow fruit or vegetable. I would recommend you eat as many of these as possible. Most of my clients still need to supplement their diet with capsules, however, as it is very hard to satisfy all nutritional requirements through food. Begin with one capsule with your evening meal for the first month and gradually increase the dose if necessary. Betacarotene is best absorbed into the body with fat or protein, so take it with the best meal of the day.

To relieve shadows and for bright sparkling eyes, I would suggest you take the following supplements:

One 50mg vitamin B complex capsule after every meal
One 1000mg vitamin C capsule after every meal
Three 15mg betacarotene capsules with your evening meal
One 50ml of Aloe Vera juice with your evening meal

For the anaemia I would recommend you take Spirulina capsules. Spirulina is a rich, highly absorbable form of iron. Begin by opening a capsule – they pull apart easily – and stir the powder into a vegetable or fruit juice at breakfast. Do the same with your evening meal. You can swallow the capsule, of course, if you are in a rush, but my advice is save these digestive juices, please.

I know most GPs recommend ferrosulphate for iron deficiencies; however, the side-effects of this are often constipation and a sore stomach as it is a very hard form of iron to digest, so I don't recommend it myself. When my daughter was pregnant and needed to supplement her iron levels with all that new blood in her body, she frequently took a highly digestible form of iron dissolved in mineral water. Its brand name is Spatone and it comes in a box of 25 individual sachets, making it easy to store and use. Available at all good health shops, it is a product of the Welsh hills and has great benefits. For those of you who enjoy the taste of liver, I would recommend you eat it twice a week for a quicker recovery as it is such a rich source of iron as well as B vitamins for the nervous system in general.

To strengthen the blood and give you lots of energy, I would recommend these supplements:

One Spirulina capsule after each meal
One 50mg vitamin B complex capsule after each meal
One Spatone sachet around breakfast as directed
One 500mg vitamin C capsule after each meal

Tiredness

You can, of course, just be plain old, plumb tuckered out. You've been doing too much and not resting enough. Or could it be that you're tired of what you're doing? Perhaps you are just tired of some of the things you do. Some people complain that they are tired, tired, tired – and yet when their friends call and ask them out, they are ready to go, go, go. I was fortunate enough to see and hear Sarah Vaughan sing in Las Vegas and one of her songs was called 'Tired'. Her opening line was 'Tired, of the life I lead', and the third line was 'Tired, counting things I need'. Sometimes our needs can be as simple as having time alone, able to do the things we want without having to consider everyone else's needs first. Oh, to be spontaneous and go with the flow. And that means you don't have to get a babysitter first! For lots of energy I would recommend lots of fun – doing something nice every day for yourself is good for you.

I would suggest you take the following supplements for increased energy and clear thinking:

> One Spirulina capsule after each meal
> One 500mg vitamin C capsule after each meal
> One 50mg vitamin B complex capsule after each meal
> One 200iu vitamin E capsule with your evening meal
> One milk thistle capsule at bedtime

Feeling sluggish and slow

I often find this unpleasant sensation is linked to a food allergy. If you think this could be a possibility then begin by varying the foods you eat. If you keep buying the same 20 items from the supermarket every week, my advice is: don't! Ask someone else to do your shopping for you. Use your local health-food shop and find organic growers who will deliver a mixed bag of fruits and vegetables to you. They deliver fresh food that's in season up to an agreed amount, of say £5, £10 or £20. That way you'll end up cooking or eating what's been delivered. These vegetables are too expensive to waste, so if they start to wilt you'll feel guilty and throw them in a soup or salad.

If you enjoy going out to eat, try new places or order different dishes at your favourite restaurants. Don't let it be that when the waiter sees you and your partner, he thinks, 'Here's the peppered steak and the chicken Kiev.' Order something different and confuse him. If you change your mind once you've ordered you can always send it back saying, 'You know we always have the steak and chicken!'

To improve your circulation I would suggest you take:

One gingko biloba capsule at breakfast
Two Spirulina capsules at breakfast
One 500mg vitamin C capsule after each meal
One 200iu vitamin E capsule with your evening meal

Moods and emotions

Do you ever feel your family could be talking about you, saying things like, 'Watch what you say to her. She's really touchy. She must be going through the change of life'? Or do they pull your leg about your up and down moods? Is it your hormones, or is it all the life changes that are going on around you? Are you feeling dissatisfied with your job or career? Is your husband or partner unsettled and talking about changing direction or early retirement? Are your children leaving home and yet still needing your financial support? What about your house? Is it falling down around you and needing repairs? Or is it too big to heat but you can't face the effort of moving and clearing out all the accumulated clutter? Coping with stress, uncertainty and change drains your body of B vitamins. Before you decide your moods are caused by your hormones, take a course of B vitamins for one month and see if your emotions level out. The water you pass will be bright yellow – that's the B2 and it's normal. If you find you are also sleeping better, it's a sure sign you were lacking B vitamins.

To relax and calm you and steady your emotions, I suggest you take:

One 50mg vitamin B complex after each meal and before bed
One Spirulina capsule after each meal
One 30ml of Aloe Vera at each meal
One 200mg magnesium tablet at breakfast
One 15mg betacarotene capsule with evening meal

How can my partner regain his zest for life and love? 14

Many couples have approached me for advice on impotence and one of the questions I'm often asked is: 'Can stress cause impotence?' The answer is yes it can, but there can also be many underlying physical causes. Diabetes can cause impotence and so can anti-depressants, beta-blockers and many other prescription drugs. Heavy metal poisoning and general ill health can lead to impotence. So the first thing I recommend is that you ask your doctor for a health check, and if you are already taking any medicine find out what the side-effects are. If you can't get enough information from your doctor you can always write to the manufacturer direct. You should – it's your health and your body.

There can be many causes for short- or long-term impotence. Could it be mental as in stress, or physical as in exhaustion and ill health? It is possible to look at impotence as a lack of physical health. Consider taking vitamin supplements to build up your health and restore your strength. Discuss your relationship and feelings with your partner, so you both understand and appreciate each other's concerns.

My area of expertise is rebuilding health and my advice will help you regain your physical well-being and put some of the zest back in your life. Let's begin by considering the factors that may have contributed to your present state of health because, yes, I do believe that impotence is a symptom of ill health and can be helped.

Your body may be sending you signals that it needs more care and attention. How many of these statements do you recognise as being true for you?

- Stressed – are you losing your sense of humour? Is anyone calling you grouchy?
- Overworked – too tired to do anything more than watch TV in the evenings.
- Overweight and snoring – putting on weight round the middle.
- Bored – losing interest in your usual hobbies. Feeling flat and lifeless, drinking more and staying longer in the pub.
- Anxious – overconcerned with small problems. Fearful of the future. Blaming others or yourself, or thinking too many 'if onlys'.
- Neglected – looking for romance and attention and feel foolish asking for tender loving care.
- Frustrated – would like to make some changes such as move to a smaller house, buy a convertible car, but concerned about rocking the boat.
- Family concerns – partner or wife menopausal, children leaving home, elderly parents needing support but no easy or quick solutions in sight.
- Physical signs of ageing – looking older than your years, losing your hair, concerned about hereditary health problems.

If you've said yes to some of the statements but have been coping well with these problems for years, why are they affecting you physically now? There is only so much a person can cope with, day in, day out. It's only natural that your body will be fed up carrying a heavy load. Something will have to give and different people react differently to this overload.

You may be thinking at this stage: 'I can't afford to lighten my load,' or 'It isn't possible for me to remove some of these problems right now.' I realise that will be true for most people, so I recommend that you give your body a boost *nutritionally* and continue with these supplements until you really feel an improvement in your state of health in general. Your body is drained at the moment.

Any person coping with these problems will only be aware of symptoms of stress on a mental level, except, perhaps, for tension in the back and neck. Your body, on the other hand, will be aware of the physical stress. Stressful circumstances are a terrible drain on your body. Let's say, for argument's sake, it takes 100 units of vitamins and minerals on an average day to keep a healthy body in good repair; during a stressful day, one hour alone will use up ten times this amount of vitamins. So although you seem on the outside to be coping with stress, your physical strength is diminishing. If you have a short-term problem such as moving house or a family member who is ill and recovers, your body will get a chance to rest and recuperate and get back to normal. But if the stresses are long term – such as business worries, redundancy fears, or something with no quick solution in sight – no matter how healthy you are or how good your diet is, the stress will wear you down. In other words, something's got to give.

Some people will display such stress through skin problems, indigestion, gall bladder problems, asthma attacks, arthritis, gout, angina or panic attacks. That's a long list but I could make it longer. I do think that all these symptoms or illnesses can be helped or prevented by extra care and vitamins. I have seen so many people totally recover from ill health and be strong and virile again. The body is always striving for balance and health. When you get an oil change in your car and the mechanic charges you for eight pints of oil, you wouldn't think of saying, 'Just use four.' You know that the car would suffer if you did. It is the same with your body. The blood coursing through your veins is lacking in nutrients and, until you replenish your body, you won't be in good shape.

All the essential vitamins, minerals and herbs needed for good health and vitality in men are:

- **Ginkgo biloba** – which is recognised for increased circulation and memory aid.
- **Ginseng** – which strengthens the body and I believe balances the energy in the body in a way similar to the effects of acupuncture.
- **Vitamin E** – essential for a strong heart and good circulation.
- **Vitamin B complex** – which strengthens the nervous system, encourages restful sleep and prevents your hair going grey prematurely.
- **Calcium and magnesium** – they calm the body and relax the muscles and I believe they are needed by the organs in your body; plus, of course, for healthy bone and joint repair.
- **Betacarotene** – which is good for eyes, hair, skin and nails and gives a feeling of well-being – and makes you good-looking!
- **Zinc and other minerals** – absolutely essential for the male reproduction system and encouraging repair and growth.
- **Vitamin C** – good for skin and repair and makes every other vitamin work twice as well.

To recover your vitality and regain your zest for life, I would recommend these supplements:

One Ginkgo capsule at breakfast
One Ginseng capsule at breakfast
One 50mg Vitamin B Complex after every meal
One Calcium, Magnesium and Zinc tablet with your evening meal
One 15mg Betacarotene capsule with your evening meal
One 200iu Vitamin E capsule with your evening meal
One 500mg Vitamin C capsule after each meal
Two 15mg Zinc tablets before bed

I believe there are many houses in Great Britain which still have original lead piping for their water supply and it is well known how toxic lead is for all of us. It's important to also consider the levels of pollutants you face at work. Paints and chemicals and even the fumes from photocopiers can have a detrimental effect on health. I am greatly concerned about the people who now spend many hours a day looking at a computer screen. Working at a VDU results in much betacarotene being drained from the body. If you need the betacarotene from one organic carrot every day to keep your eyes healthy and give you a feeling of well-being, you will need the betacarotene provided by 50 carrots every day if you spend much time at a screen or even watching television.

You are trying to relieve stress from your body so it makes sense to avoid chemicals and additives wherever possible. This in turn will naturally help your digestive process. The best foods to eat will obviously be the ones with the most nutrition, such as organic foods. Eat as much of these as you can. Include quality organic wholegrain bread, organic vegetables and fruits, organic meat and free-range eggs, nuts and seeds, especially sunflower and pumpkin seeds. A small handful of pumpkin seeds, packed with zinc, an essential mineral for all men, could be eaten once a day. Chew well. Have fresh salmon twice a week, and herring, mackerel or sardines at least once. Brewer's yeast, wheatgerm and kelp granules will also benefit your health. Drinking carrot juice every day will keep your eyes and skin healthy and give you a feeling of well-being. If it's too sweet for your taste, add a little Lea and Perrins or a few drops of Tabasco.

Take cool baths in the morning. Begin with warm water and every day gradually lower the water temperature a little. If you can manage it, have a hot and cold shower every night. A weekly massage or shiatzu treatment will also help move energy round your body and relax you.

In addition to the supplements already recommended, I would also suggest you take a 1000mg evening primrose oil capsule after your evening meal. Anyone taking these recommended vitamins will notice a huge improvement in their overall health and well-being. Take all of the tablets faithfully, for three weeks or a month, before you look for any major physical improvement – although some people will notice an improvement in their health after just a few days.

Male impotence can put a blight on any relationship, no matter how strong. A new or untested relationship can founder where there is no past steady sexual relationship to reassure both partners. It's easy for any woman to feel a failure and unattractive when her partner is impotent. If this is a new relationship and the man says it has never happened to him before, the woman may feel she must try harder, as if somehow she is part of the problem. A woman in a long-term relationship/marriage may be certain enough of herself and her husband to reassure him that it's perfectly normal, as it happens to everyone at some time.

Many people have consulted me for advice on impotence and it is most important we consider each individual's physical *and* emotional health at the same time – you can't treat one without the other.

My advice would be to take the pills I am suggesting for one month and see your health improve. Discuss your feelings with your partner and agree you will both abstain from sex for a month. During this time, however, I positively encourage you to be close in a romantic way – only, of course, if this feels right for both of you. It may be in the past that you felt being loving and romantic had to continue into a sexual act and you may have been holding back for that reason. It may be your partner expects this sequence of events as well and this is why it's important to discuss and talk through your feelings, as to what you both expect and want to happen.

To sum up, I would say take care of your physical health and make the effort to take the supplements faithfully to really see the benefits. Be loving and supportive to your partner because they might be feeling partly to blame. Don't strain for a sexual relationship too soon and nature will take its course.

Case Studies

15

I don't believe in extremes of any kind and I don't believe in telling people what to do – and that has to be a contradiction when I give advice. What I often say to a new client is that it would be so much easier for both of us if I could just take them home with me for a week and show them how they should care for themselves. I say this because I find it very hard to give sufficient advice in one meeting to change their habits and their lifestyle, yet this is what I must do if a major difference is to be made to their lives.

There has been a small percentage of my clients who kept coming to see me time after time until they succeeded in gaining their health, whatever their original problem. Most of my customers came to see me for advice, listened to my recommendations and then went off to do as they chose. I don't know the results with everyone I have advised. I do, however, know the success of those people who came back to see me week after week. Their recovery was a joint effort. I have always offered my help freely and yet it was only a determined few who persevered until they no longer needed my advice and knew how to look after their own health. I feel fulfilled and privileged that I have been allowed to help but these successes have rarely come easy. I would like to tell you about some of them. Although I have changed the names, the facts are true.

Valerie's Story

A woman brought her young teenage daughter, Valerie, to see me. The girl was suffering greatly with eczema. Her face was pale with dark circles around her eyes, which were tight and dry and red-rimmed. The skin on her face was so dry it looked as if it had been pulled tight. Her hair was thin, dry and lifeless and a mass of split ends. Her hands were covered with weeping sores which were so painful she couldn't straighten out her fingers.

I listened to Valerie's mother as she told me all the creams and lotions they had already tried, either from the doctor or chemist, and then she asked if I had a cream that would help. First I asked her to tell me about Valerie's health since birth. Once I knew more about her health in general I was able to start making my recommendations. I began by suggesting that Valerie spend seven days without eating any dairy or soya products and that she drink 30ml of Aloe Vera juice with every meal. I also recommended they buy a large 500ml tub of aqueous cream from any chemist and a large jar of evening primrose oil (EPO) 1000mg capsules. Every evening Valerie's mother was to cut open three or four of the EPO capsules and pour out this oil into a handful of the cream then gently smooth the mixture into Valerie's hands, wrists and face. I asked Valerie to keep a note of everything she ate during this week so I could get a clearer picture of what her diet was like.

They came back in a week's time. Apart from the fact that Valerie's hands weren't quite as painful, there were no other changes. My heart sank when I read what she was eating as it was mostly poor-quality convenience foods. I pointed out that most convenience foods contain milk and soya and recommended she follow a more traditional diet such as simple homemade meals, keeping the food as plain as possible. I asked Valerie to keep up her food diary and to take two evening primrose oil capsules with her evening meal. I asked her to bite into the capsules, swallow the oil and spit out the shell. So by now Valerie was now:

* on a milk- and soya-free diet
* drinking Aloe Vera juice
* swallowing 2000mg of evening primrose oil daily
* patting her skin with aqueous cream and evening primrose oil
* avoiding convenience foods
* keeping a food diary
* having as little water on her skin as possible
* taking one digestive enzyme with every meal

I saw her again the following week. Her diet hadn't improved as her mother was still feeding the whole family on convenience foods and no fresh vegetables. Until her diet included enough fresh green vegetables I recommended that Valerie take two capsules of Spirulina at breakfast every day.

Valerie's hands felt a little better so off she went to keep up the good work for another week. So Valerie was now:

* on a milk- and soya-free diet
* drinking Aloe Vera juice
* swallowing 2000mg of evening primrose oil daily
* patting her skin with aqueous cream and evening primrose oil
* avoiding convenience foods
* keeping a food diary
* having as little water on her skin as possible
* taking one digestive enzyme with every meal
* taking two Spirulina capsules a day

By this time Valerie and her parents had become avid label-readers and because they found dairy products and soya in so many ready-prepared foods it was hard to buy anything of that nature for Valerie. Her diet was improving little by little, with more fresh food being added all the time. I asked Valerie's mother to stop eating dairy and soya products herself and she agreed willingly. Her support helped Valerie a lot. We now added betacarotene and vitamin E to the list of vitamins Valerie was now taking with her evening meal. So she was now:

- on a milk- and soya-free diet
- drinking Aloe Vera juice
- taking 2000mg of evening primrose oil daily
- patting her skin with aqueous cream and evening primrose oil
- avoiding convenience foods
- keeping a food diary
- having as little water on her skin as possible
- taking one digestive enzyme with every meal
- taking two Spirulina capsules a day
- taking 15mg Betacarotene a day
- taking 200iu vitamin E a day

Often it felt like we were taking two steps forward, one step back. We would make progress and Valerie's skin would improve, but then, of course, there would be some obstacles.

Every time Valerie went swimming with the school, for example, the chemicals would irritate her skin and this would be a setback. Sometimes she would add a new food to her diet thinking it was dairy- and soya-free and then she would start to itch and realise it wasn't suitable for her. She discovered that the artificial additive flavour enhancer E621 (monosodium glutamate) in Chinese foods, Knorr cubes and some potato crisps also caused her problems. In addition, she was allergic to the additives in processed or smoked foods so she avoided them where possible. She began to drink a glass of water first thing in the morning and last thing at night and this helped cleanse her system too.

Three months after we met, Valerie's skin showed an improvement: her hands were healing and the dry patches at her elbows and behind her knees were disappearing. Her hair was stronger and healthier and growing more quickly. It took a further three months for all the changes in her diet to show through to her skin and health. At the end of six months, she was following a healthy diet, with few convenience foods, more fruit and vegetables and was drinking organic carrot juice every day, so my recommendations were:

- a milk- and soya-free diet
- drinking Aloe Vera every day
- drinking water morning and night
- 4000mg of evening primrose oil with evening meal
- 15mg of betacarotene with evening meal
- 600iu vitamin E with evening meal
- two Spirulina capsules at breakfast with organic carrot juice
- one digestive enzyme with every meal

This way of eating was now a habit and felt natural to Valerie. Her mother's health had also greatly improved as she had too enjoyed fresher foods. How did Valerie look now? Stunningly beautiful, I thought, and so did her family. Her skin was like velvet, her eyes were clear, large and sparkling and her hair was a shining, glowing mane. She was full of vibrant energy and her confidence was growing every day as she saw her reflection in the mirror.

The eczema was only an outward sign of an inner lack of vitamins and Valerie's health did improve in leaps and bounds. I discovered more about her childhood with every meeting. I believe the eczema was caused by a lack of nutritious food when she was growing up and by her mother's diet during her pregnancy (she had been on a low-fat diet). Valerie was born with a high need for essential fatty acids; while evening primrose oil will supply this, it will not do so nearly as well as mother's breast milk does, and Valerie was not breast-fed. If a baby is breast-fed until she is nine months old, the child's body can begin to produce essential fatty acids itself as well as milk-digesting enzymes. Mother's milk also contains all the essential vitamins and minerals, including vitamin E and betacarotene, plus all the nutrients Valerie's body was crying out for and which we were now providing through supplements and good healthy foods.

I enjoyed helping Valerie and her family. My advice and suggestions would have been too much for them to accept at the beginning; it was only as we followed each step and saw a gradual improvement that we had the confidence and belief to take the next step. Well done to all of us, as our success was hard earned and well deserved.

Douglas's Story

One of my clients who suffered from arthritis brought her nephew to see me as he too was complaining of joint pain. His mother had dismissed it as 'growing pains' but the discomfort had been going on for so long it could no longer be ignored as the boy was now having to take days off school and couldn't play any sport. His family knew it must be serious as he was football-mad and normally nothing would stop him playing with his friends.

I asked Douglas and his aunt to tell me about anything different that had happened the previous summer, which was when the pains had begun in earnest. Douglas and his family had moved house and the boy had to go to a new school. I wondered if that had been difficult for him as he appeared to be shy, but that didn't seem to be the problem as plenty of his old friends were at his new school too.

Douglas was suffering pains all over his body. He was having difficulty walking and felt nauseous and dizzy if he stood up for more than a few minutes. His aunt told me he had always had problems with constipation even as a baby and he now had to take laxatives every night before bed.

I asked Douglas to tell me what he ate and what his favourite foods were. He said he liked burgers, pizzas and chips, that he didn't like the taste of any vegetables and that the only fruit he liked was bananas. I asked him to keep a note of what he ate for a few days and for his mother to bring him to see me in a week's time. I recommended he take some Salusan calcium, magnesium and zinc in a liquid form as well as a 200mg magnesium tablet after his evening meal, preferably with 30ml of Aloe Vera juice. I also recommended that Douglas rest as much as possible in the seven days until I saw him again.

So Douglas was now:

- taking 30ml of Aloe Vera with every meal
- taking Salusan's calcium, magnesium and zinc drink with every meal
- taking 200mg of magnesium tablet Pharma Nord with his evening meal
- resting as much as possible

A week later he appeared with his mother who had a long list of questions for me about what might be causing Douglas's pain. I explained that I believed her son was totally drained of essential minerals and that we would now begin to rebuild his health.

This was my opportunity to find out more about what Douglas's health had been like as a baby and whether he had been breast-fed. He hadn't, so I suggested he take 2000mg of evening primrose oil a day as this would help supply him with essential fatty acids which bottle-fed babies often lack. I asked him to bite into the capsule, swallow the oil and spit out the shell.

The next step was to encourage Douglas to start eating healthier foods such as fruit and vegetables. His mother said she would stop buying convenience foods and start to cook again and that the whole family would eat that way. Next, I asked her to restrict the amount of time Douglas watched television. I explained to them that too many hours spent looking a screen, whether it's a computer or a television, will drain the body of betacarotene, the vitamin essential for good healthy bones, nails and hair and for clear, bright eyes. His mother agreed the whole family would cut down on the amount of time they spent watching television, and off they went.

So Douglas was now:

* taking 30ml Aloe Vera with every meal
* taking Salusan's calcium, magnesium and zinc drink with every meal
* taking one Pharma Nord 200mg magnesium tablet with his evening meal
* taking 2000mg of EPO with his evening meal
* resting as much as possible
* watching a maximum of one hour's television daily
* eating fresh fruit and vegetables every day.

A fortnight later, Douglas's joints were just as sore. He was also complaining of cramps in his stomach which he said he had never had before. I told him not to worry about this as it was a healthy sign that his body was now breaking down the waste that was causing constipation. Douglas agreed that he no longer experienced pain when he went to the bathroom, and he now went every day without the need for laxatives.

We added Spirulina to his diet as this multi-vitamin is easily digested and would give Douglas the extra minerals and protein needed to build good health.

What do I think caused Douglas's problems? I believe there were a number of factors. Firstly, he was not breast-fed as a baby; secondly, he hadn't been eating a good enough diet throughout his childhood; and, lastly, he played too much sport, watched too much television and had too little rest.

As a young teenager he desperately required minerals and vitamins for his growing bones and to give him enough energy to take part in the sports he enjoyed. But because his childhood diet had been so lacking in essential nutrients, these extra demands were too much for his already weakened body to cope with. Growing pains in teenagers can often be a sign that the body is crying out for extra minerals and proteins. The teenage years are also when you hear mothers say that no matter how much their children eat they are always complaining of hunger. This is the body trying to correct the imbalance – and the better the child's diet, the quicker this will happen.

It took Douglas another three months to reach peak condition and it was wonderful to see the difference in him. His diet still wasn't ideal but he knew that if he ate junk food every day he would get constipation and if he stopped taking the supplements the pain in his joints would return, so he did try to eat well. He also began taking two Spirulina

500mg capsules at breakfast stirred into a glass of Biotta carrot juice. His family made an effort to help him and kept him company by eating simple, healthy food.

Susan's Story

The following story may seem a simple one – someone being a little overweight and feeling tired and unwell. It sounds like such a common everyday problem – but that is what makes it so hard to cure. The symptoms can sound vague and not serious enough to be life-threatening and it can be difficult for overworked, exhausted doctors to be sympathetic. You may appear to be okay and still be able to work and keep going with your life and responsibilities. It may also appear that since you are still on your feet and not screaming in pain that there is nothing seriously wrong with you. Regardless of the advice of a doctor or specialist, though, you still feel unwell and it seems that the medical profession may be unable to help you further. It may be suggested to you that your problems are emotional or psychological and you may be offered a pill to help your 'mood'. Below is the story of a woman who experienced all of this and yet still had the strength to know she really was unwell and not simply unhappy. She persevered until she found a healthy answer to cure her illness.

Jane and I were friends for years and I had heard all about her sister Susan and the fact that she had been unwell for over twenty years, going from one doctor to another trying to find a cause for or solution to her ill-health.

When she and I did eventually meet, Susan explained that she always felt unwell, tired and extremely bloated. She said the doctors could find nothing wrong with her but that nevertheless she did feel ill. She knew she was about a stone overweight and the extra pounds were mostly around her middle, but that this didn't really matter to her – she just wanted to have some strength and energy to enjoy her life. She went to bed every evening about ten and slept until eight in the morning, and said that when she and her husband went out for dinner or had guests to the house it took her at least two days of resting in bed to recover her limited strength.

Because her problems had started after the birth of her first daughter and become worse after the birth of her second, I thought she might have been overloading her system with dairy products, as new mothers often do eat more milk and cheese etc than they would normally do. I asked her to avoid dairy and soya products of any kind for one month, which she agreed to do.

Susan had red hair, pale skin and blue eyes and it seems that many people with these fair colourings do not have milk-producing enzymes. Obviously not everyone with this colouring will experience discomfort digesting milk products as so much depends on what percentage of your diet is made up of other foods. Let's say in Susan's case when she was a teenager and young woman she ate a traditional Scots diet. Perhaps she had a pudding or dessert made with milk or cream once a week. She may also have had cheese once a week and then one or two bars of chocolate and one ice-cream. With the milk in her tea and coffee and something with cereal at breakfast, her total intake of dairy products in one week might have been 10 or 15 per cent of all she ate. The rest of her diet may have consisted of porridge, bread, oatcakes, sponge cake, scones, apple tart, rhubarb crumble, baked apples, bread-and-butter pudding, eggs, ham, mince, beef stew, steak and kidney, suet pudding, haddock, herring, cod, roe, kippers, lamb chops, liver and onions, soup made with ham, haugh or flank mutton, oxtail soup or chicken broth, boiled potatoes, new potatoes with skins on, boiled cabbage, mashed turnip, peas with vinegar and chips made with beef lard, soft butter lettuce, tomatoes and spring onions, jam, butter, lemon curd, apples, oranges and bananas.

None of these foods would have contained milk – even the bread-and-butter pudding would have been made with butter and whisked eggs. Butter, remember, contains no milk protein so an average amount daily will be digestible and is, I believe, good for you. So when I recommend a milk-free diet I mean no milk, cream, cheese or yoghurt – but butter is fine.

When Susan became pregnant it's likely she would have been advised to drink more milk and increase her intake of dairy products in order to boost her calcium levels. She would have heard people say that milk is good for you and gives you strong teeth and bones. That may be true if you can digest milk products; but if you can't, it follows that you won't be able to break down, extract and absorb the calcium.

Susan said that she did increase her intake of dairy foods and that this did three things. Firstly it slowed down her digestion and the absorption of essential nutrients; secondly, it filled her up and stopped her from eating other nutritious, health-giving foods; and, thirdly, she could not eliminate the waste as it wasn't digested and was lying in her stomach for too long. This led to constipation and Susan told me she suffered greatly from this common problem.

I asked her to drink as much Aloe Vera juice as possible, at least half a teacup's worth at breakfast and the same at bedtime, and to make this a habit. On her next visit she was pleased that the Aloe Vera juice and the change of diet had relieved her bloating, heartburn and stomach discomfort, but she said nothing else had improved. I asked her to continue with my recommendations and also to take a calcium, magnesium and zinc tablet after each meal, preferably with a minimum of 30ml of Aloe Vera each time to help her digestion.

On the next visit I suggested she also take two digestive-enzyme tablets with each meal and one 200mg magnesium tablet with her evening meal. So Susan was now:

- following a milk- and soya-free diet
- drinking Aloe Vera juice
- taking digestive enzymes with every meal
- taking calcium, magnesium and zinc tablets with every meal
- taking 200mg magnesium with her evening meal

We could still see only a slight improvement. Susan knew, through her sister, that I had helped many other people. She was determined to persevere and follow my advice until she became well, because she believed I really could help her.

We decided to restrict Susan's consumption of starchy foods such as rice, potatoes and pasta, and allowed her to eat only two slices of toasted bread a day until her digestion improved. I was also concerned that she might not be able to produce enough digestive juices to break down and assimilate the calcium, magnesium and zinc tablets, as minerals are always hard to digest. So she stopped the tablets and instead began to take these essential minerals in a liquid form. Salusan, who make the well-known iron tonic, Floradix, also manufacture calcium, magnesium and zinc in a fruit-juice base.

Making these two changes produced a big improvement in Susan's health and mood, and we felt we were now on the right track. Next, we added liquid vitamin E, the equivalent of 400iu, to orange juice, to be taken with her evening meal. So Susan was now:

- following a milk- and soya-free diet
- drinking Aloe Vera juice
- taking digestive enzymes with every meal
- taking liquid calcium, magnesium and zinc with her evening meal
- taking 400iu vitamin E with her evening meal
- restricting starchy food

Just adding the vitamin E made a major difference and Susan was now eliminating waste easily and naturally every morning. Constipation, thankfully, was a thing of the past.

Susan visited me once a month for four months and I saw an improvement every time we met. She lost the excess weight, her energy levels increased greatly and she felt her head was clearing and that she could now make the most of her life.

Baby Harry's Story

A young mother named Jane brought her beautiful baby boy, Harry, to see me. She was concerned that Harry wasn't thriving. He was nine months old but hadn't gained any weight since he was six months.

The baby was still being breast-fed and was eating solids three times a day. Unless he was on his mother's breast or being rocked in her arms he would be screaming with colic, pulling his legs up tight. His frequent bowel movements contained undigested food and his mother could see pieces of what she had just fed him earlier.

I began by asking Jane to keep a food diary of what she was feeding Harry and of what she herself ate, since these foods would be in her breastmilk. When I read Harry's diary I could see immediately that he was being given food that was far too hard for him to digest. When I spoke to

Jane about it, I realised she was feeding him food that had lumps in it and hadn't been puréed. Lumpy food is a sure sign that it hasn't been cooked long enough for a baby. Babies need their food well cooked, sieved if necessary, and then puréed.

I asked Jane to begin to feed Harry as though he were four months old and just starting solids and she willingly agreed. I recommended very basic foods such as organic carrots, well cooked and then puréed, and the same with organic dessert apples. I also suggested she prepare Harry's porridge from jumbo organic oats, cooking it slowly, which he could have for breakfast and then later in the day as a pudding. I also discovered that Jane was using a microwave to heat Harry's food and when I pointed out its potential side-effects, she agreed to stop this.

As Jane's diet was mostly a vegetarian one, and she ate a great deal of dairy and soya products, I was concerned that this might be one of the reasons behind Harry's severe colic. Jane agreed to add fish to her diet and to restrict her intake of dairy products and soya. To assist in the elimination of these foods from her system, I asked her to take 30ml of Aloe Vera with each meal and two Spirulina capsules each time she ate, thus supplementing her diet with vitamins and protein. I also recommended she take 3000mg of EPO with her evening meal and 200iu of vitamin E at the same time.

So Jane was now:

- following a milk- and soya-free diet
- eating fish every day
- taking 30ml of Aloe Vera at mealtimes
- taking two 500mg capsules of Spirulina after each meal
- taking 3000mg of EPO with her evening meal
- taking 200iu of vitamin E with her evening meal

I also asked Jane to give her son at least 2000mg of EPO every day by cutting open the capsules and pouring the oil directly into his mouth. It's good to do this at bath time as any extra oil can be massaged into the baby's skin.

The next step was to explain to Jane how important it was to keep Harry warm and always to wrap him up well when she was taking him out in the pram or car, ensuring that he had a hat and scarf on. This really was a case of wrapping the baby in cotton wool. I wanted to make sure Harry's body wasn't using up valuable energy just to keep warm. I wanted all his energy to go into making him strong and healthy as quickly as possible.

Imagine that Harry has three meals a day. On the days he is kept warm and cosy his body can use all the nutrients and goodness in his food to build strong bones and a healthy body. If there is a day when Harry is underdressed for the weather and is cold then firstly he won't be able to digest his food properly, and secondly it may take the energy or goodness from one or even two of his meals simply to maintain the temperature required to keep his body on an even keel. So instead of all three meals being used to provide strength and health, it may be that only one can be given over to growth.

We wanted Harry to thrive as quickly as possible and so we had to take extra care. His mother did everything I asked and within three days the little boy was free from colic – although he was still passing undigested spinach in his bowel movements from food eaten five days earlier. His mother was pleased to tell me he was now smiling at everyone all the time.

Harry was now:

- on a milk- and soya-free diet
- only eating food that had been puréed
- having 2000mg of EPO daily

- being kept warm at all times
- eating nothing that had been microwaved
- being breast-fed on demand
- sleeping in his mother's bed for warmth and comfort
- taking Kindervital Multi-Vitamin Drink by Salusan

I continued to see Harry and his mum for another six months and we all learned a lot during that time. Jane freely admitted that her own mother had brought her up in a 'casual' way and that she, Jane, just didn't know what was best for Harry. But she was so eager to learn. As Harry began to thrive and we could see we were on the right track with his foods and keeping him warm, Jane's confidence and pride in being a mother began to grow and I felt she now had the strength to consider taking some more healthy steps.

I asked her not to give Harry any food from tins or cartons – glass jars were best – and obviously only to buy organic foods. I asked her always to dilute Harry's fresh fruit juices and vegetable juices with an equivalent amount of boiled water. I told Jane not to let Harry sleep or spend any time in a room with a computer in it, whether on or off, and not to let him sleep with his head near an electric socket. She was also to ensure that everything he wore and slept in was made of 100 per cent natural fibres – cotton, wool, linen and silk – and that she was to keep him away from manmade fibres where possible.

Jane told me that Harry's buggy was brand new, but when I saw it I realised that the little boy was facing away from his mother, and she couldn't see him either when they went out for a walk. I asked Jane if she knew anyone who had an old-fashioned Silver Cross pram that she could borrow. It took another six weeks before she found one and

I felt a lot happier when I saw Harry lying in it. He was much higher off the pavement than in his buggy. The Silver Cross was less draughty and gave more protection from the wind, and the little boy could see his mother. Because of all this, and because he could now stretch out straight, he slept better and more soundly when they were out walking.

Jane took the buggy when it wasn't practical to use the Silver Cross – such as visiting the supermarket – but when she saw how much more comfortable her baby was in the big pram, with no crying or discomfort, she asked her husband to do all the shopping, perhaps on his way home from work, and kept the use of the buggy to a minimum. The outcome was a happier baby, happier mother, and therefore a happier father.

One of the final things Jane and I discussed as Harry grew stronger and healthier was their family holiday. My heart sank when she said they planned to spend two weeks in Florida with her sister's family. I was greatly concerned that a long-haul flight like this would badly affect Harry's health. I asked Jane to postpone any lengthy flights until her son was at least five years old, and preferably older. Instead I recommended she restrict Harry's flying to one round trip a year, and only a short hop of an hour or so each way, and never to a polluted city. Three months later I received a postcard from the island of Jersey saying Harry loved playing on the beach.

Harry's daily diet was now as follows:

Breakfast: Half a peeled and sliced organic apple or pear or banana. Half a teacup of Biotta organic carrot juice with boiled warm water added to make up a full cup and with one Spirulina 500mg capsule opened and the powder stirred into the juice. (The powder has no taste at all, and some mothers mash it into their baby's porridge or pudding once a day instead of into the juice.) One or two tablespoons of toasted wheatgerm with one or two tablespoons of stewed or puréed apples with one or two teaspoons of cream. One organic egg either scrambled or in an omelette. One slice of organic bread, either plain or toasted.

Mid-morning: a biscuit, fruit and juice.

Lunch: half a cup of homemade soup. Small piece of fish or chicken with mashed potatoes and carrot and onion.

Mid-afternoon: as morning.

Tea or dinner: a small portion of shepherd's pie. A cup of homemade rice-pudding made from organic or goat's milk, with raisins.

What should I eat for a healthy figure?

16

I think it's important that before you read the 14 menus I make clear again my thoughts behind the advice which follows. These suggestions are made only to encourage you to pay more attention to what you eat. As I said at the beginning of the book, when you were growing up your family may not have eaten well and you may still be living that way today. I also previously mentioned that I would so much like to be able to show people how to shop for, prepare and enjoy good meals that would lead to good health for them and their family.

Although at present organic food is the more expensive option, I think the benefits it gives more than outweigh the cost of eating cheaper, poorer quality products.

If you saw me shopping and cooking you would see I buy and cook only with the best quality olive oil and organic butter. I am very particular about the quality of the food I buy and eat. I think it's worth the amount of effort I put in – I know it is the reason why I have such good health and why I really do have so much energy and optimism. I feel good every morning when I wake up and this is because my body has been nourished and given the amount of care and attention it needs.

I've met a lot of overweight, tired, lethargic and depressed students who have lived on junk food for two years or more, and although they all seem to appreciate the idea that 'it's not good to live on junk food', they don't seem to follow the thought through to 'it's not good to live on junk food because it doesn't have the nutrients or vitamins needed for good health and brain energy'. These are the things students need most (apart from a gold American Express card and a doting rich grandmother).

We are coping with so much pollution in our environment it really is essential to eat the best, nutritious food available. I go to a lot of effort to find and buy bread and bakery products free of soya of any kind, and that usually means I have to buy fresh bread every day. I make sure the oatcakes I buy are made only with oats, and if I buy anything which contains vegetable oil I want to know exactly what kind of oil it is – I want to be certain I am not eating anything that has been genetically modified. I always buy free-range eggs, but I prefer organic free-range eggs when I can find them, as I am concerned that even free-range farmers may be giving their chickens genetically modified feed. Some poultry offered for sale bears the label 'corn-fed' but this corn could be genetically modified.

I buy goat's and ewe's cheeses from Ian Mellis (see the mail-order address list at the end of the book). Because I don't eat a lot of cheese, and because goats and ewes are not commercially fed, it doesn't have to be organic. About three quarters of the fruits and vegetables I eat are organic, though.

If I were your hostess for a day I would prepare and cook the following for you. For breakfast: either a glass of Biotta organic carrot juice or two organic carrots and one apple freshly juiced; a bowl of organic porridge, made with jumbo oats, with organic brown sugar and organic cream, and a tablespoon of Bemax toasted wheatgerm on top; an omelette, cooked with olive oil, made with two free-range or organic eggs, a chopped organic tomato and a small handful of grated goat's cheese; organic bread toasted or warmed in the oven, spread with organic butter and organic jam; and tea or coffee, finishing with an organic apple.

Lunch would be a piece of fresh haddock or cod, dipped into a beaten egg, coated with organic breadcrumbs and shallow-fried in a mixture of butter and olive oil with two cloves of crushed garlic, plus an organic green salad on the side; then some gingerbread or fruit loaf with organic butter and tea or coffee.

The evening meal would start with homemade organic carrot soup, followed by roasted free-range chicken with yellow peppers and chillis, served with organic boiled potatoes, mashed with organic butter and organic cream and organic broccoli; dessert would be organic apple crumble and organic ice-cream and then coffee and Belgian chocolates.

This is the way I prefer to cook and eat. I am not able to eat like this every day, only about half the time. The rest of the time it can be a combination of either a good breakfast, perhaps hardly any lunch and then the evening meal in a restaurant – although I will enjoy this food I wouldn't expect it to be nutritious. For that I've got to cook at home.

DAY 1

BREAKFAST

1 egg – boiled, fried, poached or scrambled
2 slices of brown toast with butter and marmalade or jam
Tea (with full cream milk) or coffee (with cream)
*As much fresh fruit as you would enjoy, either before or after
  breakfast*

LUNCH

Turkey or ham with salad in a brown bread sandwich
Apple and pear
Tea (with full cream milk) or coffee (with cream)

DINNER

Haddock – poached, grilled or fried in olive oil, butter and garlic
Mashed potatoes and green beans
Home-made apple or rhubarb crumble (see recipe on p.160)
Tea (with full cream milk) or coffee (with cream)

SUPPER

*Oatcakes with pâté (many different pâtés available: black olive,
  mushroom, chicken liver, spicy bean, tuna, smoked salmon,
  duck)*

DAY 2

BREAKFAST

Grilled bacon
2 slices brown toast with butter and marmalade or jam
Tea (with full cream milk) or coffee (with cream)
As much fresh fruit as you would enjoy, either before or after
breakfast

LUNCH

Tuna or prawn salad sandwich
Apple and kiwi fruit
Tea (with full cream milk) or coffee (with cream)

DINNER

Home-made hamburger (see recipe on p.160)
oven chips or boiled potatoes, unpeeled
mixed green salad with an olive oil and fresh lemon dressing
Carrot cake
Tea (with full cream milk) or coffee (with cream)

SUPPER

Crackers with hummous

DAY 3

BREAKFAST

2 slices of cold ham or cold meat of your choice
2 slices brown toast with butter and marmalade or jam
Tea (with full cream milk) or coffee (with cream)
As much fresh fruit as you would enjoy, either before or after
   breakfast

LUNCH

Tuna or prawn salad sandwich
Banana and grapes
Tea (with full cream milk) or coffee (with cream)

DINNER

Chicken – roasted with skin on (see recipe on p.161)
Broccoli and carrots
Sponge cake or gingerbread and butter
Tea (with full cream milk) or coffee (with cream)

SUPPER

Toast and pâté

DAY 4

BREAKFAST

Bacon and egg or kippers
2 slices brown toast with butter and marmalade or jam
Tea (with full cream milk) or coffee (with cream)
As much fresh fruit as you would enjoy, either before or after
  breakfast

LUNCH

Baked potato with filling of your choice plus salad
Orange and banana
Tea (with full cream milk) or coffee (with cream)

DINNER

Spaghetti bolognese (see recipe on p.161)
Mixed green salad
Apple pie or Eccles cake
Tea (with full cream milk) or coffee (with cream)

SUPPER

Shortbread fingers

DAY 5

BREAKFAST
1 egg – boiled, fried, poached or scrambled
2 slices of brown toast with butter and marmalade or jam
Tea (with full cream milk) or coffee (with cream)
As much fresh fruit as you would enjoy, either before or after breakfast

LUNCH
Roast beef or pork sandwich
Pear and banana
Tea (with full cream milk) or coffee (with cream)

DINNER
Fish pie (see recipe on p.162)
Peas, preferably fresh but frozen will do
Gingerbread and butter
Tea (with full cream milk) or coffee (with cream)

SUPPER
Cheese or ham toastie

DAY 6

BREAKFAST

1 egg – boiled, fried, poached or scrambled
2 slices brown toast with butter and marmalade or jam
Tea (with full cream milk) or coffee (with cream)
As much fresh fruit as you would enjoy, either before or after
  breakfast

LUNCH

Chicken salad sandwich
Crisps
Pear and orange
Tea (with full cream milk) or coffee (with cream)

DINNER

2 lamb chops, grilled
Mashed potatoes (with butter and milk)
Cabbage – boiled, or chopped thinly and stir-fried
Apple pie or rhubarb crumble with cream or ice-cream
Tea (with full cream milk) or coffee (with cream)

SUPPER

2 shortbread fingers

DAY 7

BREAKFAST

Eggs and cornbread fried or toasted (see recipe on p.163)
Tea (with full cream milk) or coffee (with cream)
As much fresh fruit as you would enjoy, either before or after breakfast

LUNCH

Roast beef sandwich
Apple and kiwi
Tea (with full cream milk) or coffee (with cream)

DINNER

Tagliatelle carbonara (see recipe on p.164)
Green salad with oil and lemon dressing
Tiramisu or Italian panettone
Tea (with full cream milk) or coffee (with cream)

SUPPER

Sardines on toast

DAY 8

BREAKFAST
1 egg – boiled, fried, poached or scrambled
2 slices of brown toast with butter and marmalade or jam
Tea (with full cream milk) or coffee (with cream)
As much fresh fruit as you would enjoy, either before or after
*   breakfast*

LUNCH
Ham sandwich
Grapes and bananas
Tea (with full cream milk) or coffee (with cream)

DINNER
Skinless chicken breast dipped in beaten egg, rolled in
*   breadcrumbs and shallow-fried in olive oil*
Boiled potatoes with skins on
Broccoli
Carrot cake
Tea (with full cream milk) or coffee (with cream)

SUPPER
Cheese or ham toastie

DAY 9

BREAKFAST
Bacon and egg or kippers, either grilled or poached in a little water
2 slices brown toast with butter and marmalade or jam
Tea (with full cream milk) or coffee (with cream)
As much fresh fruit as you would enjoy, either before or after breakfast

LUNCH
Tuna salad sandwich
Sponge cake
Fresh fruit
Tea (with full cream milk) or coffee (with cream)

DINNER
Haggis, neeps and tatties
Fruit salad with cream or ice-cream
Tea (with full cream milk) or coffee (with cream)

SUPPER
Hummous with pitta bread

DAY 10

BREAKFAST

Sausages or bacon with potato scone
Tea (with full cream milk) or coffee (with cream)
As much fresh fruit as you would enjoy, either before or after
    breakfast

LUNCH

Chicken salad sandwich
Kiwifruit and pear
Tea (with full cream milk) or coffee (with cream)

DINNER

Quiche Lorraine (see recipe on p.165)
Green salad with oil and lemon dressing
Fresh fruit
Tea (with full cream milk) or coffee (with cream)

SUPPER

Pâté and toast

DAY 11

BREAKFAST

2 slices of cold ham or cold meat of your choice
2 slices brown toast with butter and marmalade or jam
Tea (with full cream milk) or coffee (with cream)
*As much fresh fruit as you would enjoy, either before or after
    breakfast*

LUNCH

Tuna or prawn salad sandwich
Banana and grapes
Tea (with full cream milk) or coffee (with cream)

DINNER

Beef stew (see recipe on p.163) and vegetables
Cornbread (see recipe on p.163)
Apple pie
Tea (with full cream milk) or coffee (with cream)

SUPPER

Hummous and crackers

DAY 12

BREAKFAST
1 egg – boiled, fried, poached or scrambled
2 slices brown toast with butter and marmalade or jam
Tea (with full cream milk) or coffee (with cream)
As much fresh fruit as you would enjoy, either before or after
breakfast

LUNCH
Roast beef or corned beef salad sandwich
Apple and pear
Tea (with full cream milk) or coffee (with cream)

DINNER
Fried lemon sole – washed, dipped in plain flour, then fried in a
mixture of butter and olive oil at a medium heat
Gruyère potatoes (see recipe on p.167)
Mangetouts or Brussels sprouts
Fresh fruit salad
Tea (with full cream milk) or coffee (with cream)

SUPPER
Oatcakes and pâté

DAY 13

BREAKFAST

Sausage or bacon
2 slices of brown toast with butter and marmalade or jam
Tea (with full cream milk) or coffee (with cream)
As much fresh fruit as you would enjoy, either before or after breakfast

LUNCH

Hard-boiled egg and salad and oatcakes
or egg mayonnaise sandwich-filler
Apple and banana
Tea (with full cream milk) or coffee (with cream)

DINNER

Skinless chicken breast dipped in beaten egg, rolled in breadcrumbs and shallow-fried in olive oil
New potatoes, boiled
Broccoli or mangetouts
Gingerbread and butter
Tea (with full cream milk) or coffee (with cream)

SUPPER

Small omelette

DAY 14

BREAKFAST

1 egg – boiled, fried, poached or scrambled
2 slices of brown toast with butter and marmalade or jam
Tea (with full cream milk) or coffee (with cream)
As much fresh fruit as you would enjoy, either before or after
*   breakfast*

LUNCH

Tuna or prawn sandwich
Banana and orange
Tea (with full cream milk) or coffee (with cream)

DINNER

Spaghetti and meatballs (see recipe on p.166)
Fruit
Tea (with full cream milk) or coffee (with cream)

SUPPER

Cheese or ham toastie

The recipes – some simple home-cooked meals

17

Apple or Rhubarb Crumble

> 2–3 large Bramley cooking apples, peeled and sliced, or 4–5 stalks
> of rhubarb, chopped into one-inch pieces
> 1½ cups plain flour
> 2oz butter
> 2 tbsp brown sugar

Cook the apples or rhubarb until tender (about 8 to 10 minutes) in just enough water to cover the fruits, with brown sugar to taste, depending on the tartness of the fruit. Put the cooked fruit into a buttered casserole dish.

Rub the flour and butter between your fingers until they form a crumbly mixture; stir in the sugar. Spread the mixture on top of the cooked fruit. Bake in a preheated hot oven (gas mark 6) for 30 minutes until browned.

Hamburgers

> Allow 4oz of mince per person

Place meat in bowl, add finely chopped onion and the yolk of one egg (per 8oz of mince) and seasoning to taste. Mix well and form into patties. Fry in a little olive oil, turning once. For quicker cooking, make into two small burgers.

Roast chicken

One fresh chicken breast (with skin on) per person
½ onion, chopped
1 medium carrot, sliced
1 stalk celery, roughly chopped
1 clove garlic

Wash chicken and place in casserole with skin uppermost. Add the vegetables and garlic clove. Pour in a little cold water until chicken is half covered. Drizzle one tablespoon of olive oil over each piece of chicken, then salt. Cook uncovered for 30 minutes in preheated medium oven.

Spaghetti Bolognese

Allow 4oz of mince per person
2 tbsp olive oil
1 onion, chopped
1 large carrot, chopped
2 or 3 stalks of celery, chopped
1 or 2 garlic cloves
½ tsp mixed Italian herbs
1 jar of passata
1 tin of chopped tomatoes

Warm most of the olive oil in a large saucepan, then add the beef a little at a time. Keep stirring until the meat is browned and cooked, which will be 5 to 10 minutes. Then add the onion, carrot, celery and garlic.

Fry these vegetables in the remaining oil in the middle of the meat for two minutes, then add the mixed herbs and seasoning to taste. Stir through, add the passata, tomatoes and a cup of water. Simmer for at least 1 hour, 2 if possible.

Fish Pie

(serves 2–3)
2 fresh haddock fillets (about 6oz each)
4 medium potatoes, peeled and sliced
1 carrot, sliced
1 cup milk (in which to poach fish)

For the white sauce:
1 knob of butter
2 tsp plain flour
1 cup of milk

To poach the fish:
Place the fish in a small frying pan and cover with milk. Bring to boil and simmer for 2 to 3 minutes then turn off heat.

For the topping:
Put the potatoes and carrots in a saucepan of cold water. Bring to boil and cook for 20 minutes until soft. Drain and mash with butter and a little milk.

To make the white sauce:
Melt a little butter in a small saucepan on a low heat, adding the flour a little at a time and mixing to a smooth paste. Once all the flour has been added, add the milk very gradually, stirring constantly, so the paste thins out to a pouring sauce consistency.

To assemble the pie:
Gently fold pieces of the fish into the potato and carrot mixture, adding the milk if needed. Place in a buttered casserole dish and pour over the white sauce. Sprinkle grated cheese or breadcrumbs on top, and bake in a hot oven (gas mark 6) for 25 minutes until brown on top.

Cornbread

1½ cups cornmeal or maize
½ cup plain flour
1 tsp baking powder
½ tsp salt
2 tsp sugar
2 eggs, beaten
1 cup milk
2 tbsp olive oil
water as needed

Mix all the dry ingredients together in a large bowl. Then add the eggs beaten with the milk and stir well. Finally add the olive oil and enough water very gradually to give a thick, pouring batter.

Pour the mixture into a greased and floured baking tin (a small loaf tin would be best, or a size 8 or 9 round tin) and bake in a medium oven for about 20 to 25 minutes until risen and brown on top.

Beef Stew

1lb cubed beef
2 potatoes, peeled and quartered
2 carrots, scraped and sliced
2 onions, peeled and quartered
2 stalks celery, sliced
2 cloves garlic, peeled and crushed
2 tbsp olive oil, more as needed
½ cup plain flour
1 tsp Marmite for stock flavouring (or use 1 or 2 additive-free
    FRIGG stock cubes, available from health-food shops)
salt and pepper

Put the flour in a small paper bag and add a handful of beef cubes. Close and shake the bag. Put these floured cubes to one side and continue until all cubes are coated. Do the same with the vegetables.

Heat the oil in a frying pan. When it's hot enough, it will shimmer. Brown a few cubes of meat at a time and transfer them to a large pot. Continue this way until all the meat is browned. Add more oil to pan and repeat this process with the vegetable pieces. Add them to the large pot. Add seasoning to taste.

Place the Marmite or stock cubes in a jug and dissolve with two cups of hot water. Pour over the meat and vegetables. Bring to boil, reduce heat to simmer and cook for approximately 90 minutes. You may need to add more water or stock as it cooks.

Tagliatelle carbonara

8oz uncooked tagliatelle

For the sauce:
3 or 4 rashers of bacon, chopped
2 eggs
2 egg yolks
2 tbsp cream
2 tbsp Parmesan cheese
salt and pepper

Place the pasta in boiling water, with one tsp of olive oil added, and bring to the boil. Reduce heat and cook for time it says on the packet.

Meanwhile, fry the chopped bacon in olive oil until crisp. Remove from the heat. Drain the cooked pasta and add to the frying pan on top of the bacon. Beat the two eggs and two egg yolks together and then add cream to this mixture. Stir into the pasta and bacon in pan. Add seasoning to taste. Serve with Parmesan cheese.

Quiche Lorraine

For the shortcrust pastry:
8oz plain flour
2oz butter, chopped into small pieces
pinch of salt
4 tbsp cold water

For the filling:
4 eggs
2 slices bacon, chopped finely
2oz grated cheese – Cheddar or Edam
½ cup of milk

You can, of course, buy ready-made pastry, but to make your own, put the flour in a bowl and add the butter. Rub the butter and flour between your fingers until the butter disappears and the mixture resembles breadcrumbs.

Sprinkle the cold water evenly over the surface and stir in with a round-bladed knife until the mixture begins to stick together in lumps. With one hand gather the dough together to form a ball. One of the secrets of successful pastry is to touch it very little in order to keep it as cold as possible.

Roll out the pastry. Line a greased and floured baking tray with it.

Place dried beans or pulses of any kind on top of the uncooked pastry, enough to cover base evenly, and bake in a hot oven for 20 minutes. This is called 'baking blind' and it's just to stop the pastry rising. Prebaking it this way means you won't have a soggy base when it's filled and cooked at the next stage.

Let the pastry cool for ten minutes or more and then prepare the filling.

Fry the bacon in olive oil for 3 or 4 minutes, until cooked but not crisp, and turn off the heat. Beat the eggs and milk together and pour into the pastry base, then add the bacon and cheese to the quiche. Sit the case on a baking tray and then bake in a hot oven for about 20 to 30 minutes until the eggs are set and the top is slightly browned.

Meatballs

2 tbsp olive oil or more as needed
½ lb minced beef
½ lb minced pork
1 carrot, grated
1 onion, finely chopped
2 cloves of garlic, peeled, crushed and finely chopped
2 egg yolks
½ cup plain flour
½ tsp mixed herbs
1 jar of pasta sauce
1 cup of water
salt and pepper

Place the meat and vegetables in a bowl and add herbs and seasoning to taste. Then add the egg yolks, mix together and form the mixture into small balls. Roll lightly in the flour.

In a frying pan, heat the oil until shimmering. Add the meatballs, reduce the heat a little, and keep turning until cooked all over.

Meanwhile, warm the sauce and water in a separate pan.

If you have any carrot or onion left over, you can add it to the sauce. When warmed through, transfer the cooked meatballs to the sauce and simmer for at least 10 minutes before serving.

Potatoes, leeks and Gruyère

3 medium potatoes, thinly sliced
1 medium leek, cleaned and chopped
100g Gruyère cheese
1 quantity white sauce (see recipe on p.162)
salt and pepper

Arrange the potato slices and leek in a greased ovenproof dish. Break the Gruyère into pieces over the vegetables, add seasoning to taste and cover with the white sauce.

Bake in a medium hot oven for about 40 to 45 minutes or until the top is browned.

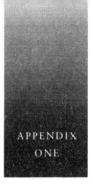

Supplements

Aloe vera

Hundreds of scientific papers describe the active benefits of Aloe Vera gel taken internally or applied externally to skin and hair. These include Aloe as:

- *a natural cleanser and tissue penetrator*
- *a bactericidal – a strong antibiotic, even when diluted*
- *viricidal, when in contact for long periods*
- *fungicidal*
- *an anti-inflammatory*
- *an antipuritic – it stops itching*
- *a nutritional product – provides vitamins, minerals and natural sugars*
- *an antipyretic – reduces heat of sores*
- *anaesthetises tissue, relieving pain associated with joint problems*
- *dilates capillaries, increasing circulation*

Aloe Vera is extremely safe and has no known side-effects.

Vitamin C

Unlike most other mammals, human beings lack the ability to synthesise vitamin C. During stress, infection and certain other conditions, there is an increased need for vitamin C which our metabolism cannot supply.

The primary role of vitamin C is in the formation of collagen, which is important for the growth and repair of body tissue cells, gums, blood vessels, bones and teeth.

Some of the other well-known properties of vitamin C are:

- heals wounds, burns and bleeding gums
- accelerates healing after surgery
- helps in decreasing blood cholesterol
- aids in preventing many types of viral and bacterial infections
- acts as a natural laxative
- lowers the incidence of blood clots in the veins
- aids in the treatment and prevention of the common cold
- reduces effects of many allergy-producing substances

B complex

The B group of vitamins is a collection of essential nutrients that have certain characteristics in common. These water-soluble vitamins, whilst chemically distinct from each other, are closely interrelated when they work in the body. For example, folic acid and vitamin B12 metabolisms are closely connected; vitamin B2 is required for the activation of B6; and B3 can be manufactured from other dietary agents, provided there is adequate B6. So it is usual that when a deficiency of one of the B vitamins is suspected, a B Complex is given. A summary of the complex is as follows:

- **Vitamin B1 (Thiamin)** plays a part in energy production and carbohydrate metabolism
- **Vitamin B2 (Riboflavin)** plays a crucial role in the formation of a number of enzymes that are mainly

found in the liver

- **Vitamin B3 (Nicotinic Acid and Nicotinamide)** *plays an important role in the formation of certain enzymes that are involved in the transport of hydrogen*
- **Vitamin B5 (Pantothenic Acid)** *plays a crucial role in many of the reactions involving carbohydrates, fats and amino acids*
- **Vitamin B6 (Pyridoxine)** *plays an important role in the metabolism and its constituent amino acids*
- **Vitamin B12** *is involved in the regeneration of red-blood cells and also in the proper utilisation of fats, carbohydrates and protein*
- **Folic Acid** *is used to improve lactation; protect against intestinal parasites and food poisoning; act as an analgesic for pain, and increase appetite (if you are run-down)*
- **Paba** *has important sun-screening properties and can help restore your hair to its natural colour*

Spirulina

Spirulina is a microscopic freshwater plant which blooms naturally on Lake Chad in the Sahara Desert and other freshwater lakes. This organic superfood, with its remarkable energising and rejuvenating properties, was used historically by the Aztecs who sustained themselves (sometimes solely) on Spirulina wafers.

This vegetable multi-vitamin contains over a hundred synergistic nutrients. It is very easily digested, allowing its concentrated nutrients, enzymes and living essences to be absorbed into the bloodstream without the momentous loss of energy incurred in the digestion of ordinary foods.

Spirulina contains:

- **Vitamins:** *Betacarotene (pro-vitamin A), Thiamin (B1),*

Riboflavin (B2), Niacin (B3), Pyridoxine (B6), Cyano-
cobalamin (B12), Folic Acid, Biotin, Pantothenic Acid
(B5), Inositol, Bioflavanoids (Rutin), Tocopherol (E)
* **Minerals:** Calcium, Phosphorus, Potassium, Sodium,
Iron, Magnesium, Zinc, Copper, Chromium, Selenium,
Manganese
* **Amino Acids:** histidine, isoleucine, lysine, methionine,
phenylalanine, threonine, tryptophan, valine, alanine,
arginine, aspartic acid, cystine, glutamic acid, Glycine,
proline, serine, tyrosine
* **Pigments:** phycocyanin, chlorophyll, carotenoids.
* **Nucleic Acids:** RNA (ribonucleic acids), DNA
(deoxyribonucleic acids)

Vitamin E

Vitamin E, along with vitamin C, is one of the most popular vitamin
supplements and has from time to time been recommended as a
treatment for almost every conceivable medical condition – such
are the properties of this remarkable vitamin.
It is fat soluble and its absorption from the intestine depends upon
effective fat digestion and absorption. So diseases of the stomach,
pancreas and liver can produce a vitamin E deficiency. A deficiency
can also cause the destruction of red-blood cells, muscle
degeneration, some anaemias and reproductive disorders.
There are many benefits to taking a vitamin E supplement. These
include:

* keeping you looking younger by retarding cellular
ageing due to oxidation
* supplying oxygen to your body to give you more
endurance
* protecting your lungs against air pollution by working
with betacarotene

- *preventing and dissolving blood clots*
- *alleviating fatigue*
- *preventing thick scar formation externally*
- *accelerating healing of burns*
- *working as a diuretic, it can lower blood pressure*
- *aiding the prevention of miscarriages*

Betacarotene

Betacarotene is a fat-soluble vitamin which your body converts into vitamin A as required, thus avoiding the potential toxicity of taking too much vitamin A.

Among many of betacarotene's properties, the most important and well-known is in relation to eye function. Betacarotene is necessary to prevent drying of the eye and corneal changes; also, the normal function of the retina, the part of the eye involved with vision, and particularly the function of the light-sensitive areas of the eye are dependent on there being sufficient betacarotene.

Betacarotene is also involved in a number of other bodily functions, apart from the counteraction of night-blindness and weak eyesight. These include:

- *the building of resistance to respiratory infections*
- *a reduction in the duration of diseases*
- *helping keep the outer layers of your tissues and organs healthy*
- *promoting growth, strong bones, healthy skin, hair teeth and gums*
- *helping in the removal of age spots*
- *helping treat acne, impetigo, boils, carbuncles and open ulcers*
- *aiding in the treatment of emphysema and hyper-thyroidism*

172

Recommended products

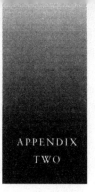

Supplements (available from quality health-food shops)

Bioforce herbal products:
Hypericum (St John's Wort)
Saw Palmetto Complex
Menosan (for women)
Pharmanord Coenzyme Q10, Selenium and magnesium tabs
Salusan calcium/magnesium/zinc drink, magnesium drink and
  Kindervital (vitamins for children) drink
Solgar Advanced Cartenoid Complex, B50 Complex and
  calcium/magnesium/zinc tablets
Bumbles royal jelly (500mg capsules) (distributed by Power Health)
Quest digestive enzymes and evening primrose oil (100mg capsules)
Lanes vitamin E (200, 500 and 1000iu capsules)
Lifestream Aloe Vera juice
ESI Aloe Vera juice (distributed by Health Imports) and EPO liquid
  (bottled)
Natural Options spirulina (500mg capsules), Aloe Vera juice and EPO
  capsules
Regina royal jelly (fresh in phials – for a special occasion!)
Spatone produce a highly absorbable natural form of iron in mineral
  water (contained in individual daily sachets)
Natures Answer – herbal tinctuals – alcohol-free (distributed by
  Health Imports)

Food Products (available from quality health food shops)

Green & Blacks for all chocolate products, ice-cream, hot chocolate
Bemax toasted wheatgerm (a good source of B vitamins)
Biotta or **Evernat** organic carrot and other juices
Rice Dream organic rice milk drink
Whole Earth organic peanut butter, organic marmalade and jams, organic baked beans
Zest pasta sauces (all are additive-free, some are organic)

Own-brand Supplements

The following supplements have been formulated and manufactured to my own specification:
Spirulina
Enzyme Digest
Speedslim™
These supplements contain only natural herbal ingredients, and are easy to digest.

For further information on these products, or for a list of stockists please telephone or write:

Laura Ackerman
713 Great Western Road
Glasgow
G12 8QX
Telephone 0141 339 2669

Recommended mail-order suppliers

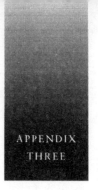

Ian Mellis Cheese Monger – *Shops in Edinburgh (2) and Glasgow. Ian Mellis specialises in British and Irish farmhouse cheeses, maturing these to perfection in his own curing rooms.*
I.J. Mellis Cheese Monger, Unit 81a, Albion Business Centre, Albion Road, Edinburgh EH7 5QZ, telephone 0131 661 4440, fax 0131 656 9114.

Jenners Department Store – *Luxury hampers, caviar, smoked oysters. 48 Princes Street, Edinburgh, EH2 2YJ, telephone 0131 225 2442.*

Loch Fyne Oyster Bar – *Famous for smoked salmon, kippers, pâtés and, of course, oysters. They have a huge mail-order list which they will happily post, fax or e-mail to you.*
Loch Fyne Oysters Limited, Clachan, Cairndow, Argyll PA26 8BL, telephone 01499 600234, e-mail loch_fyne.co.uk.

Macsween of Edinburgh – *Family business specialising in the production of traditional haggis, the national dish of Scotland. You can receive haggis, vegetarian haggis, fruit pudding, mealy pudding or their delicious black pudding by mail order.*
Macsween of Edinburgh, Dryden Road, Bilston Glen, Loanhead, Edinburgh EH20 9LZ, telephone 0131 440 2555, fax 0131 440 2674, e-mail haggis@macsween.co.uk.

The Teviot Smokery, *Water Gardens and Coffee Shop – situated in the beautiful Scottish Borders between Jedburgh and Kelso, this place is famous for salmon, trout, succulent eels and wild game of every kind. Usually open six days a week (closed Sunday), except*

from between 1 April and 30 September, when open seven days.
The Teviot Smokery, Kirkbank House, Eckford, Kelso, Roxburghshire
TD5 8LE, telephone 01835 850253, fax 01835 850293.

The Ubiquitous Chip – Restaurants, bars and wine shop. Sells
organic wines.
The Ubiquitous Chip, 8 Ashton Lane, Glasgow G12 8SJ, telephone
0141 334 5007.

Raeburn Fine Wines – This excellent wine merchant sells organic
wines from all over the world. The owner is a very knowledgeable
wine buff who will personally advise you.
Raeburn Fine Wines, 23 Comely Bank Road, Edinburgh EH4 1DS,
telephone 0131 343 1159.

Tombuie Smokehouse – Situated in the heart of Perthshire. Sells
wonderful smoked bacon and other meats.
Tombuie Smokehouse, Aberfeldy, Perthshire PH11 2JS, telephone
01887 820127, fax 01887 829625.

The House of Bruar – Marvellous food hall. Mail-order hampers.
The House of Bruar Ltd, by Blair Atholl, Perthshire PH18 5TW,
telephone 01796 483236, fax 01796 483218.

Scotland's Larder – Beautiful restaurant with Aga, shop, cookery
demonstrations and mail-order service. Close to St Andrews,
overlooking the Firth of Forth. The owner and (excellent) chef,
Christopher Trotter, will help you to source unusual foods or
products. Very committed to Scottish produce.
Scotland's Larder, Upper Largo, Fife KY8 6EA, telephone 01333
360414, fax 01333 360427.